Clinician's Guide to Adult ADHD Comorbidities

Joseph Sadek

Clinician's Guide to Adult ADHD Comorbidities

Case Studies

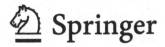 Springer

Joseph Sadek, MD, B.Sc. Pharm., MBA, FRCPC
Diplomat American Board of Psychiatry and Neurology (ABPN)
Associate Professor
Department of Psychiatry
Dalhousie University
Halifax
Nova Scotia
Canada

ISBN 978-3-319-39792-4   ISBN 978-3-319-39794-8   (eBook)
DOI 10.1007/978-3-319-39794-8

Library of Congress Control Number: 2016953205

Printed on acid-free paper

This Springer imprint is published by Springer Nature
The registered company is Springer International Publishing AG Switzerland

I want to give my sincere thanks to my wife Irene and my children Joseph and Maryanne who were extremely supportive during the journey of producing this book.

Biography of Dr. Joseph Sadek

Dr. Sadek is an Associate Professor of Psychiatry at Dalhousie University and the clinical and academic leader, Nova Scotia Hospital, Mayflower Unit. He is also the medical director of the Atlantic ADHD Center in Dartmouth, Nova Scotia, Canada

Dr. Sadek is a Diplomat of the American Board of Psychiatry and Neurology (DABPN) and fellow of the Royal College of Physicians and Surgeons of Canada (FRCPC). In addition to his medical degree (1990), Dr. Sadek also holds a pharmacy degree (B.Sc. Pharm. 1986) and an MBA from St. Mary's University, Halifax. He also completed a 1-year research training program at Harvard Medical School and obtained the certification of the Global Clinical Scholars Research Program (GCSRP) with commendation. He completed his psychiatry residency training at Dalhousie University.

Dr. Sadek served as the head of the Neurosciences professional competency unit for the Dalhousie Medical School. He started the first public adult ADHD clinic in Nova Scotia in 2007. He is heavily involved in both the undergraduate and postgraduate teaching and has published a book called *Clinician's Guide to ADHD*, second edition in 2013. Dr. Sadek has several peer-reviewed articles and received several quality awards for his work. He served as the vice president of the Canadian ADHD Resource Alliance (CADDRA) and created the CADDRA ADHD institute in 2012.

Dr. Sadek is currently the chair of the Suicide Prevention Task Force for the Province of Nova Scotia. He was also a member of the Dalhousie University, Senate. He was the chair of the Capital District Health Authority (CDHA) Investigation sub-Committee and served in other committees including: Credentials Committee, Undergrad Curriculum Committee, Senate Discipline Committee of Dalhousie University, District Medical Staff Association, CDHA (vice President), Psychiatry Medical Staff Association (President), Mortality and Morbidity Committee (chair for 7 years), and Research Ethics Board of CDHA from 2002 to 2011.

Dr. Sadek received the Mental Health Program Quality Council Certificate of Excellence Award for commitment to quality review (2012) and Mental Health Program Quality Council Certificate of Excellence Award for development and implementation of suicide risk assessment form (2012).

Contents

Introduction

There is a need for a clear and concise approach to a complex disorder such as attention deficit hyperactivity disorder (ADHD). Understanding the diagnosis and management of ADHD is incomplete without understanding comorbidities and how to manage them.

This guide uses a case-based approach to explain how to diagnose and manage ADHD in presence of comorbid disorders. Despite the complexity of the topic, each case brings a unique prospective on ADHD patients. The consistent approach in describing the cases allows clinicians to think of broader differential diagnosis and then come to a clear impression and plan.

Each case is supported by literature review on different areas such as epidemiological data, etiology, morbidity, diagnosis, and management approaches.

This book captures some important disorders that co-occur with ADHD such as depression, bipolar mood disorders, substance use disorders, and personality disorders.

One chapter is dedicated to review malingering and ADHD and another discusses the recent findings about the link between obesity and ADHD.

The cases are practical and relevant for clinicians and the literature review is extensive and clear.Several resources are included in this book to help clinicians expand their knowledge around ADHD comorbidities. They include questionnaires, rating scales, web sites, and ample references.

This guide is intended for educational purposes only. There are different areas in the field of ADHD that were not captured in this guide and readers are encouraged to continue to update their knowledge regularly.

ADHD and Borderline Personality Disorder (BPD)

1

1.1   The Case of Leah Lee

Objectives
1. Review the epidemiology and etiology of ADHD and BPD
2. Describe some of the key similarities and differences between borderline personality disorder and ADHD
3. Recognize the importance of identifying comorbid personality disorder in adults with ADHD
4. Understand the management approaches for patients with BPD and ADHD
5. Recognize the challenges in treatment of ADHD in presence of BPD

1.2   Leah Lee

- Leah is a healthy 25-year-old single female who lives alone in Portland, Main. She works at a grocery store.
- *Patient complaint at the office of her family doctor:* "I am very depressed and anxious. I need a note to stay off work for the next 3 months. She said I need a change".
- *History of present illness and review of systems*:
- Leah started this job 6 month ago. She feels that the store manager appreciates her work but the other cashiers hate her and want her to leave. She said none of them mentioned that but her feelings are certain about that. She said that customers are very nice to her because they can tell she is very stressed out. She has been making some carless mistakes at work and the assistant manager mentioned that to her briefly, so she decided to go on sick leave.
- Mood symptoms: patient reported hourly mood changes that range from irritability to depression or sudden happiness. She also reported lack of motivation and procrastinating. She is trying to lose weight, despite having ideal body weight, so she watches what she eats but does not restrict her food intake. When she was a

© Springer International Publishing Switzerland 2017   1
J. Sadek, *Clinician's Guide to Adult ADHD Comorbidities*,
DOI 10.1007/978-3-319-39794-8_1

teenager she used lots of laxatives but she does not use them anymore. No binging nor purging behavior. She describes long lasting feelings of low self-esteem but her energy and appetite are good. She enjoys outdoor activities, watching movies, and playing video games. She has no suicidal intent or plans but she threatens suicide if she does not get a note to stay off work. When stressed she scratches her arm. Her attention and concentrate have been described as poor as long as she remembers. Denies feelings of guilt and her sleep is poor with frequent awakening in the middle of the night. She thinks that most of her symptoms started when she was a teenager and never left.

- Anxiety symptoms: Patient has chronic worry about people not liking her and not being the center of attention despite her good looks and ideal body weight. She can control her worries but feels restless all the time. Negative screening for phobia, obsessive compulsive disorder (OCD), PTSD, and panic episodes.
- Alcohol and substance use: Leah will binge drink weekly and on weekends she drinks 12–24 beers until she is drunk. She is open to trying street drugs when offered in parties. She used cocaine and LSD 4 years ago but did not use them since. Currently she uses small amounts of weed when she cannot sleep. She started drinking and using drugs at age 14. She does not see alcohol use as a problem. She describes it as helpful and fun.
- Psychosis: Leah feels that people talk about her behind her back. "They do not like me and stare at me" she said and she stopped interacting with many of them. Screening for hallucinations and delusions was negative.
- *Past psychiatric history:* Multiple short admissions (less than 1 week) to hospital over the past 9 years. She was referred for outpatient mental health but she never showed up. She has been on multiple SSRI/SNRI antidepressants, which she stopped after few weeks because of intolerable side effects, or lack of effectiveness in her opinion.
- *Medical history:* No known allergy. Healthy. Had one abortion at age 15.
- *Family history*: Leah has one brother and one sister. Parents divorced when she was 4 years old. Leah's paternal grandparents abused drugs and alcohol. Her mother and brother have been diagnosed with depression and anxiety. Her sister suffers from ADHD.
- *Developmental, personal and social history*: Her mother smoked cigarettes while pregnant with Leah, but consumed neither street drugs nor alcohol. Normal delivery and no delay in developmental milestones. She was described as hyperactive child who was accident prone. During elementary school she received average marks and was often defiant with teachers. Teachers frequently commented that she does not finish her home work, does not listen in class, and talks too much that she distracts other kids. She hated school but was able to get along well with other children. She failed grade 6 after a year of sexual abuse by her step father. Her mother found out and divorced him. He was charged and had a jail sentence for abusing Leah and seven other children in the area. Leah feels that she never received affection and love as a child.

School performance improved in her final year of high school after having a very supportive guidance counselor. She had difficulty paying attention in class and found mathematics very challenging that she always needed tutoring and extra support. Leah's report cards mentioned consistently that she cannot pay attention in class and that she is easily distracted. Leah said that she has difficulty sitting down to do her homework and she cannot finish more than few pages of any book that she starts. Her mother convinced her to go to university so she did after a significant struggle but dropped out after the first semester. Leah describes significant difficulties sustaining her attention in lectures. Her mind always wonders. Her car and room are very messy and disorganized. She avoided the assignments in university because it requires focusing and that was the same during school but her mother had to force her to sit down and complete her work then.

On the positive note, Leah is very artistic and has won a number of awards for her works of art and dance performances. Has two close friends, although she says, "some days I feel they hate me but I do not want them to leave me. They do not like that I interrupt them all the time but I do not care."

- *Sexual history*: A history of multiple chaotic sexual relationships, but currently single. History of casual sexual encounters without the use of adequate birth control. Had an abortion at age 15 and became pregnant after a one-night stand then. She started promiscuous sexual behavior at age 13 and had over 50 partners since then. None of her relationships lasted more than 6 months. She also had some relationships with females but did not continue them. Leah mentioned that she was raped at age 17 by her boyfriend.
- *Occupational history*: She worked in call centers. Has lost a number of jobs for chronic lateness. Quit last job impulsively after feeling that her manager hates her.

Collateral History Patient consented to talking to her mother Linda who confirmed the following.

She had to force Leah to sit down and complete her homework because she avoids doing it. Leah lost so many items during elementary school that she had to go to school frequently to try to find them. These items included her jacket, her gym shirts, her books, and her homework. Leah is easily distracted and much disorganized. She was very talkative and loud but now she does not talk nearly as much. Leah does not listen because of day dreaming all the time.

She has severe mood swings and could destroy the furniture when she is angry. Leah binge drinks and can spend all her work money on pay day then comes to her mother to borrow money. She used to binge and purge a lot more as a teenager. Now she watches what she eats. Mom is very concerned with her alcohol and street drug use.

At this point Leah was referred to see a psychiatrist.

1.3   Summary of the Findings and Management of This Patient

After reviewing the collateral history, interviewing the patient and completing the assessment, the psychiatrist listed the following disorders in the initial diagnostic impression:

ADHD inattentive type, alcohol use disorder, borderline personality disorder, and history of eating disorder NOS.

The psychiatrist ordered blood work including TSH that all appeared within normal limits. He asked the patient to complete several rating scales and questionnaires. He explained his diagnostic impression to Leah including all the symptoms of borderline personality disorder. He provided her with education and insight. Leah was delighted to understand her symptoms and was relieved to hear that her problems are not diagnosed as depression since she tried so many antidepressants in the past with no success. She agreed to start DBT psychotherapy program and was also started on a stimulant medication (lisdexamfetamine 30 mg) in the morning. She was also prescribed melatonin 5 mg at bedtime that improved her sleep. The benefits and risk of medications and the possible alternative treatment were explained to her and she felt agreed to start the treatment. She was referred back to her family doctor after starting the DBT program and tolerating the medication well. She was able to continue to work, and 1 year after starting treatment for ADHD and BPD her symptoms were much improved and she was able to continue to work.

Literature Review Questions
Discuss the epidemiology and comorbidity of ADHD and borderline personality disorder (BPD)?

Attention deficit/hyperactivity disorder (ADHD) is seen as a neurodevelopmental disorder starting before the age of 12, according to the DSM-V. More than 50 % of the children suffering from ADHD still displayed clinically relevant symptoms when reaching adulthood, with a high degree of psychiatric comorbidities [1], among which borderline personality disorder (BPD) is encountered more often than expected by chance [2, 3].

ADHD is characterized by a persistent pattern of inattention and/or hyperactivity/impulsivity that can interfere with or reduce the quality of social, academic, or occupational functioning. However, when diagnosing ADHD in adults, it is important to note that the expression of key symptoms can change with age. In particular, hyperactivity and impulsiveness tend to decline with increasing age, whereas inattention tends to persist [4, 22]. Symptoms such as hyperactivity may change into feelings of inner tension or restlessness [5], which can then be mistaken as signs of anxiety or depression.

In some cases, the diagnosis of ADHD can be difficult, particularly when the disorder is severe and presents with mental health symptoms that may mimic those of other mental health disorders such as borderline personality disorder (BPD). At times, symptoms that overlap with those of ADHD and can lead to inaccurate diagnosis and/or management.

Failure to recognize a comorbid personality disorder in an adult with ADHD may lead to the wrong assumption of treatment failure if pharmacotherapy for ADHD does not bring about adequate clinical and functional improvement. In addition, individuals with ADHD and comorbid borderline personality disorder may need additional interventions, such as dialectical behavioral therapy, to address serious symptoms such as self-injury and distorted perception (Lieb et al.).

Comorbidity rates between ADHD and borderline personality disorder (BPD) are well documented in the literature. The overlap may seem unusually strong. For example, Philipsen et al. [3] found only 16 % comorbidity of BPD with ADHD. On the other hand, a more recent study [6] reported a number as high as 38 %.

Both ADHD and borderline personality disorder have indistinguishable comorbidity rates for substance use, anxiety and eating disorders, and very similar levels of cyclothymia, which may point to mood lability as a common denominator of these disorders [7].

Some data suggest that ADHD patients without symptoms of BPD are less predisposed to be nervous, tense, and insecure than ADHD patients with symptoms of BPD. That finding is in line with the characterization of BPD in terms of emotional instability. They also scored significantly higher on the character dimensions self-directedness and cooperativeness than did the other patients and, in fact, showed normal character development [8].

List some of the different hypothesis that are proposed to account for the comorbidity between ADHD and BPD?

1. The comorbid disorders do not represent distinct entities but rather are the expression of phenotypic variability of the same disorder.
2. Each of the comorbid disorders represents distinct and separate clinical entities.
3. The comorbid disorders share common vulnerabilities, either genetic (genotype), psychosocial (adversity), or both.
4. The comorbid disorders represent a distinct subtype (genetic variant) within a heterogeneous disorder.
5. One syndrome is an early manifestation of the comorbid disorder (i.e., ADHD is an early manifestation of a mood disorder).
6. The development of one syndrome increases the risk for the comorbid disorder (i.e., ADHD increases the risk for borderline personality disorder). Investigations of these issues should help to clarify the etiology, course, and outcome of ADHD [9].

What are the diagnostic symptoms criteria of borderline personality disorder?

According to DSM V [10], patient has to have a long-standing pattern that started in early adulthood that causes significant impairment in function and meets 5 of the following criteria:

- An intense fear of abandonment, even going to extreme measures to avoid real or imagined rejection or abandonment.
- A pattern of unstable intense relationships, sometimes seeing things as black and white or using splitting as a defence.

- Rapid changes in self-identity or self-image that include shifting goals and values.
- Periods of stress-related paranoia and loss of contact with reality, lasting from a few minutes to a few hours. It can be described as micro psychotic or dissociative experience.
- Impulsive and risky behavior, such as, reckless driving, sex, spending sprees, binge eating or drug abuse, or gambling.
- Suicidal threats or behavior or self-injury, often in response to fear of separation or rejection.
- Significant and wide mood changes or swings that can happen within the same day, lasting from a few hours to a few days, which can include intense happiness, irritability, or anxiety.
- Long-standing feelings of emptiness.
- Inappropriate, severe anger episodes or difficulty controlling anger, such as frequently losing temper, being sarcastic or bitter, or having physical fights.

Describe some of the key similarities and differences between borderline personality disorder and ADHD?

Both disorders are chronic, disabling, and impairing conditions that are pervasive across many situations and might share impulsivity as a common symptom (ADHD combined type and hyperactive-impulsive type). ADHD has childhood onset or early adolescent onset while BPD has early adult/adolescent onset; signs in childhood in some cases. Some key differences: inattention is not a core feature of BPD; however, frantic efforts to avoid real or imagined abandonment is one of the core feature of BPD. Recurrent suicidal behavior is a core feature of BPD but not ADHD. Hourly mood fluctuation is a core feature of BPD but some affective lability might be found in ADHD [11].

Some neuroimaging studies suggest that for ADHD and BPD, there may be some shared neurobiological dysfunction, thus a degree of overlap may exist in underlying brain dysfunctions, as well as in symptomatology. For instance, there may be dysfunctions of the prefrontal cortex, a core region for attentional mechanisms and impulse control, and in the orbitofrontal cortex, a core region for impulsivity and emotional control (Broome [12]).

Anger expression and aggression are reported to be higher in comorbid BPD and ADHD ([13]).

Why is it important to recognize a comorbid personality disorder in an adult with ADHD?

Failure to recognize a comorbid personality disorder in an adult with ADHD may lead to the wrong assumption of treatment failure if pharmacotherapy for ADHD does not lead to adequate clinical and functional improvement.

In addition, individuals with ADHD and comorbid borderline personality disorder may need additional interventions, such as dialectical behavioral therapy, to address serious symptoms such as self-injury and distorted perception [14,15].

What are some of the helpful tips for managing borderline patients in primary care setting?

- Learn about common clinical presentations and causes of undesirable behavior.
- Validate the patient's feelings by naming the emotion you suspect, such as fear of abandonment, anger, shame, and so on, before addressing the "facts" of the situation, and acknowledge the real stresses in the patient's situation.
- Avoid responding to provocative behavior.
- Schedule regular, time-limited visits that are not contingent on the patient being "sick."
- Set clear boundaries at the beginning of the treatment relationship and do not respond to attempts to operate outside of these boundaries unless it is a true emergency.
- Make open communication with all other providers a condition of treatment.
- Avoid polypharmacy and large-volume prescriptions of potentially toxic medications (including tricyclic antidepressants, cardiac medications, and benzodiazepines).
- Avoid prescribing potentially addicting medications such as benzodiazepines or opiates. Inform patients of your policies regarding these medications early in the treatment relationship so they are aware of your limits.
- Set firm limits on manipulative behavior while avoiding being judgmental.
- Do not reward difficult behavior with more contact and attention. Provide attention based on a regular schedule rather than being contingent on behavior [16].

What are the key clinical recommendations in adults with BPD and ADHD?
Psychotherapy is the primary treatment for BPD. Principals of dialectic behavior therapy (DBT) may be helpful in adult ADHD patients as an adjunct to medications.

No fully evidence-based pharmacotherapy exists for the core BPD symptoms although some medications may be effective for individual symptom domains, e.g., impulsivity.

Treatment of ADHD should be considered when treating comorbid personality disorders. Treating the core syndrome of ADHD may result in better functioning, less distress, more control over behavior, and possibly will have more engagement and benefit from psychotherapy [11].

Give examples of psychotherapeutic approaches for patients with BPD?
Examples of empirically studied treatments for BPD include: dialectic behavior therapy (DBT), mentalization-based therapy, transference-focused psychotherapy, and general psychiatric management.

Several types of these psychotherapies have a manual and require therapists to undergo extensive training, to be self-aware and have access to therapy or consultation by other colleagues to avoid burnout.

DBT is an outpatient treatment involving group and individual therapy and considered as an effective treatment for BPD. DBT focuses on teaching the patient how to regulate emotions, manage self-destructive feelings and behaviors, tolerate distress, and develop interpersonal effectiveness and ability for reality testing. It uses different techniques over at least 1 year, including acceptance and mindfulness. It has been found to reduce self-harm and suicidality in addition to lowering health care costs and utilization of emergency department and inpatient admission.

Mentalization-based therapy is another group and individual psychotherapy. The goal of treatment is focused on helping the patient to "mentalize" or understand the mental state of oneself and others and to think before reacting.

Transference-focused psychotherapy is an individual, twice-weekly therapy derived from psychoanalysis. It is focused on transference (feelings of the patient projected onto the therapist), and is among the more difficult techniques to learn.

General psychiatric management is a once-weekly psychodynamic therapy. It focuses on the patient's interpersonal relationships and can also include pharmacotherapy and family therapy. This is the most available and easiest to learn. In general, effective treatment requires the patient's active involvement and commitment [16].

Other examples include cognitive behavioral therapy (CBT), dynamic deconstructive psychotherapy (DDP), and interpersonal therapy for BPD (IPT-BPD) [17].

Is there any evidence for mindfulness based interventions in ADHD and BPD?

Although only few studies have investigated the effectiveness of mindfulness training in ADHD (many of which showing methodological limitations), some researchers do suggest that mindfulness may be useful in ADHD interventions. Mindfulness means paying attention and being aware of the experiences occurring in the present moment, and some authors argue that mindfulness training is associated with improved attention systems and self-regulation, and that it therefore fosters those skills that are underdeveloped in individuals with ADHD [18].

What are the management difficulties in patients with comorbid ADHD and BPD that are related to BPD?

Patients with BPD can be difficult to manage for a number of reasons. For one they often elicit countertransference reactions in the treating physician which can lead to the over- or underprescription of pharmaceuticals. Patients with BPD may struggle with accurately assessing response to ADHD medications. As such it is important to rely on objective measures when gauging response to treatment. It is also very important to maintain appropriate boundaries at all times with BPD patients. When patient expectations are not met, they may react with feelings of abandonment, rage, disappointment, or devaluation [19].

What is the general approach to pharmacotherapy for BPD?

Cochrane review of 27 trials stated that the current evidence from randomized controlled trials suggests that drug treatment, especially with mood stabilizers and second-generation antipsychotics, may be effective for treating a number of core symptoms and associated psychopathology, but the evidence does not currently support effectiveness for overall severity of borderline personality disorder. Pharmacotherapy should therefore be targeted at specific symptoms [20].

What are the literature recommendations for pharmacological therapy for patients with ADHD and BPD?

There appears to be very limited data in relation to treatment of patients with comorbid ADHD-BPD. One study suggested that treating comorbid BPD–ADHD subjects with methylphenidate, as opposed to not treating them, was associated with greater improvements in several dimensions, which include, ADHD severity, impulsiveness, and the tendency to express anger, but the study had only 14 female subjects [21].

Other reviewers argued that, while many patients with BPD receive "off label" medications, no robust evidence of efficacy exists for pharmacotherapies in relation to "the core BPD symptoms of chronic feelings of emptiness, identity disturbance and abandonment".

Patients with BPD may have some tendencies to misuse or abuse controlled substances, therefore careful prescribing should take place particularly for short acting stimulant medications [22].

With regard to the noradrenergic systems, clonidine treatment, which has been reported to effectively reduce impulsivity and hyperactivity in children and adolescents with ADHD, may also reduce aversive inner tension and the urge to self-harm in patients with BPD [23].

One author suggests that treating the core syndrome of ADHD may result in better functioning, less distress, and more control over behavior and possibly will have more engagement and benefit from psychotherapy [11, 24, 25].

References

1. Kessler RC, Adler L, Barkley R, Biederman J, Conners CK et al (2006) The prevalence and correlates of adult ADHD in the United States: results from the National Comorbidity Survey Replication. Am J Psychiatry 163:716–723
2. Bernardi S, Faraone SV, Cortese S, Kerridge BT, Pallanti S, Wang S, Blanco C (2012) The lifetime impact of attention deficit hyperactivity disorder: results from the National Epidemiologic Survey on Alcohol and Related Conditions (NESARC). Psychol Med 42:875–887
3. Philipsen A, Limberger MF, Lieb K, Feige B, Kleindienst N, Ebner-Priemer U, Barth J, Schmahl C, Bohus M (2008) Attention-deficit hyperactivitydisorder as apotentiallyaggravat-ingfactorinborderlinepersonalitydisorder. Br J Psychiatr 192:118–123
4. Biederman J, Mick E, Faraone SV (2000) Age-dependent decline of symptoms of attention deficit hyperactivity disorder: impact of remission definition and symptom type. Am J Psychiatry 157:816–818
5. Kooij SJ, Bejerot S, Blackwell A et al (2010) European consensus statement on diagnosis and treatment of adult ADHD: The European Network Adult ADHD. BMC Psychiatry 10:67
6. Ferrer M, Andión O, Matalí J, Valero S, Navarro JA, Ramos-Quiroga JA et al (2010) Comorbid ADHD in borderline patients defines an impulsive subtype of borderline personality disorder. J Personal Disord 24:812–822
7. Perugi G, Toni C, Maremmani I, Tusini G, Ramacciotti S et al (2012) The influence of affective temperaments and psychopathological traits on the definition of bipolar disorder subtypes: a study on bipolar I Italian national sample. J Affect Disord 136:e41–e49
8. Van Dijk FE, Lappenschaar M, Kan CC, Buitelaar JK et al (2012) Symptomatic overlap between attention-deficit/hyperactivity disorder and borderline personality disorder in women: the role of temperament and character traits. Compr Psychiatry 53(1):39–47
9. Davids E, Gastpar M (2005) Attention deficit hyperactivity disorder and borderline personality disorder. Prog Neuropsychopharmacol Biol Psychiatry 29(6):865–877
10. American Psychiatric Association (2013) Diagnostic and statistical manual of mental disorders, Fifth Edition (DSM-5). American Psychiatric Publishing, Arlington
11. Asherson P, Young AH, Eich-Höchli D, Moran P, Porsdal V, Deberdt W (2014) Differential diagnosis, comorbidity, and treatment of attention-deficit/hyperactivity disorder in relation to bipolar disorder or borderline personality disorder in adults. Curr Med Res Opin 30(8): 1657–1672

12. Broome MR, He Z, Iftikhar M, Eyden J, Marwaha S (2015) Neurobiological and behavioural studies of affective instability in clinical populations: a systematic review. Neurosci Biobehav Rev 51:243–254
13. Prada P, Hasler R, Baud P, Bednarz G, Ardu S, Krejci I, Nicastro R, Aubry JM, Perroud N (2014) Distinguishing borderline personality disorder from adult attention deficit/hyperactivity disorder: a clinical and dimensional perspective. Psychiatry Res 217(1–2):107–114
14. Mao AR, Findling RL (2014) Comorbidities in adult attention-deficit/hyperactivity disorder: a practical guide to diagnosis in primary care. Postgrad Med 126(5):42–51
15. Lieb K, Zanarini MC, Schmahl C, Linehan MM, Bohus M (2004) Borderline personality disorder. Lancet 364(9432):453–461
16. Dubovsky AN, Kiefer MM (2014) Borderline personality disorder in the primary care setting. Med Clin North Am 98(5):1049–1064
17. Stoffers JM, Völlm BA, Rücker G, Timmer A, Huband N, Lieb K (2012) Psychological therapies for people with borderline personality disorder. Cochrane Database Syst Rev 8:CD005652
18. Schmiedeler S (2015) [Mindfulness-based intervention in ADHD]. Z Kinder Jugendpsychiatr Psychother 43(2):123–131
19. Gabbard G, Wilkinson S (2000) Management of counter transference with borderline patients. Jason Aronson Inc. ISBN-10: 0765702630
20. Lieb K, Völlm B, Rücker G, Timmer A, Stoffers JM (2010) Pharmacotherapy for borderline personality disorder: cochrane systematic review of randomised trials. Br J Psychiatry 196(1): 4–12
21. Prada P, Nicastro R, Zimmermann J, Hasler R, Aubry JM, Perroud N (2015) Addition of methylphenidate to intensive dialectical behaviour therapy for patients suffering from comorbid borderline personality disorder and ADHD: a naturalistic study. Atten Defic Hyperact Disord 7(3):199–209
22. Larsen H, Dilshad R, Lichtenstein P et al (2011) Developmental trajectories of DSM-IV symptoms of attention-deficit/hyperactivity disorder: genetic effects, family risk and associated psychopathology. J Child Psychol Psychiatry 52:954–963
23. Philipsen A, Richter H, Schmahl C, Peters J, Rüsch N, Bohus M, Lieb K (2004) Clonidine in acute aversive inner tension and self-injurious behavior in female patients with borderline personality disorder. J Clin Psychiatry 65(10):1414–1419
24. Philipsen A (2006) Differential diagnosis and comorbidity of attention-deficit/hyperactivity disorder (ADHD) and borderline personality disorder (BPD) in adults. Eur Arch Psychiatry Clin Neurosci 256(Suppl 1):i42–i46
25. Philipsen A, Feige B, Hesslinger B et al (2009) Borderline typical symptoms in adult patients with attention deficit/hyperactivity disorder. Atten Deficit Hyperact Disord 1:11–18

ADHD and Malingering

2

Objectives
1. Review historical data on malingering in medicine
2. Review epidemiological data on malingering and ADHD
3. Review the utility of soma available tools in detecting malingering in ADHD
4. List some of the clinical tips for detecting malingered ADHD?

2.1   The Case of Martin Miles

Identification MM is a 20-year-old male student who is currently in his second year of university. He lives in a small apartment with two roommates close to the university campus.

Chief Complaint Patient referred himself to the university health clinic complaining of poor attention.

He said that he was diagnosed at age 8 with ADHD and he was prescribed medications but his parents did not allow him to take medications then. He said that his attention is very poor and all he wants is a prescription of Dexedrine.

History of Present Illness Patient said that he has been failing courses and he cannot focus since the beginning of this year. He filled several ADHD rating scales that he found online and brought them to the office. He selected the most severe ratings for all symptoms of inattention on all the scales.

Alcohol and substance use screening: patient said he drinks couple of beers during weekends. He said he only tried cocaine few times and but started using weed regularly for the past 18 months.

Mood disorder screening: He reported good mood, good energy and appetite, no suicidal thoughts and no previous attempts. His sleep is great but his concentration and attention is very poor. He enjoys reading novels, business books, and history books. He said he can read for days. No active symptoms of mania.

© Springer International Publishing Switzerland 2017
J. Sadek, *Clinician's Guide to Adult ADHD Comorbidities*,
DOI 10.1007/978-3-319-39794-8_2

Anxiety screening: MM is very worried about his academic performance and his finances. He said that anxiety is new. He can control his anxiety. Screening for phobia, PTSD, OCD, and panic disorder was negative.

Psychosis screening: denied hallucinatory experience. He has no delusions. His behavior and speech are organized and his thought process is clear and organized.

Past Psychiatric History He said his only encounter with mental health was at age 8 when he was diagnosed with ADHD.

Medical History Patient has no known drug allergies. He had asthma as a child and used puffers but no longer requires medication. He had few broken bones when he was a teenager after several fights.

Family History Patient has one older sister who is currently in jail. She was involved in a break and enter incident and has a recent history of cocaine use after getting involved with a boyfriend who has a significant criminal record. His mother had depression and his father is alcoholic and has been out of his life for the past 3 years. He said that his father left the house one day and moved in with one of his sister's friends who was much younger than him. The family stopped talking to him since then.

Personal and Social History Patient was born in Vancouver, BC, Canada. He said he is not aware of any problems in his mother's pregnancy. His delivery was normal and he had no developmental delays.

He said his father was authoritarian and controlling and was never supportive of him nor his sister. He tried to get the approval of his father by doing well in school but his father never acknowledged that.

He is close to his mother and talks to her frequently. MM has several close friends and had 4 previous girlfriends since age 16. He has been with his current girlfriend for 1 year but he cheated on her twice. He laughed when he mentioned that.

School History MM enjoys playing sports and he played basketball in his high school team. When asked about school, he said that school was a source for stress for him. He was bullied for several years and teachers did not like him. He has never failed any grades or subjects and was never diagnosed with specific learning disability. Academically he was on the top of the class.

Work History He worked in fast food restaurants but was fired from the past 2 jobs and he said he is not sure why.

The following conversation took place about ADHD symptoms:

Doctor: How often do you have problems paying attention to details or making careless mistakes in school or at work?
Patient: All the time.
Doctor: Can you give me an example?

Patient: I miss reading the questions on the exams so I give the wrong answer.

Doctor: When did that start happening?

Patient: Since last year.

Doctor: How often are you distracted by things around you (e.g., while doing school work, during lectures or classes)?

Patient: All the time

Doctor: What distracts you?

Patient: Hearing my professor's voice during economics lecture.

Doctor: Can you explain?

Patient: I hate my economic professor, so as soon as he speaks, I get distracted.

Doctor: Does this happen in other classes?

Patient: No. Not really.

Doctor: Does noise or movement distracts you?

Patient: No. I am good with that.

Doctor: How often do you avoid tasks that require mental effort (e.g. doing school assignments or preparing reports)?

Patient: All the time. I did not hand any assignment this year.

Doctor: When did that problem start?

Patient: All my life since I was 3 years old.

Doctor: But you did not have to do any assignment then?

Patient: But I was diagnosed with ADHD.

Doctor: How often do you have difficulty listening to what people say to you, even when they are speaking to you directly?

Patient: All the time.

Doctor: But you have been very good with me here today. Listening to my questions.He started getting very angry.

Patient: You see all I am here for is to get my prescription. I am not here to answer your useless questions.

Doctor: I have to ask questions to understand the symptoms.

Patient: Fine. Just do it.

Doctor: How often do you lose things or cannot find them such as keys, paperwork, wallet, bank cards, or mobile phone?

Patient: All the time. I lost 5 phones this year.

Doctor: This year???

Patient: May be in the past 2 years. ....ok. Do you understand?

Doctor: How often do you have difficulty staying focused while doing some tasks that do not interest you (e.g., during lectures or lengthy readings or boring work)?

Patient: All the time. I cannot read anything.

Doctor: How often do have difficulty staying organized (e.g., work is disorganized, room is messy, fail to meet deadlines, poor time management)?

Patient: I am very organized. This is not my problem.

Doctor: How often do you have trouble finishing projects or school work (e.g., start tasks but quickly lose focus and leave things incomplete)?

Patient: I can finish things. This is not my problem.

Doctor: How often do you have problems remembering things such as appointments, paying bills, or in other daily activities?

Patient: All the time. My memory is really bad.

Doctor: Do you forget things that happened recently or things that happened many years like in junior high school or names of your high school teachers?

Patient: Things that happened many years ago like my teachers' names.

Doctor: So you can remember appointments and recent events?

Patient: Yes.

He denied hyperactivity impulsivity symptoms.

He gave permission to call his mother and he was scheduled to come in one week.

Collateral Information from His Mother Mom said that he was never diagnosed with ADHD and was very smart in school. She said that his roommates have been using street drugs and he got involved with them in the past year. She is worried that he wants medications to them because he has been calling her lately asking for money. She is very concerned that he started failing his university courses but he did very well in his first year. She said school reports until he finished high school were commenting on his excellent achievements and never mentioned inattention or inability to finish school work.

She never had to ask him to do his homework and he was always organized.

Impression and Plan MM reports a recent change in his attention which is not characteristic of ADHD. Collateral information reveals that the information he provided is inaccurate and he never had the diagnosis of ADHD nor the symptoms. At this point, bringing the patient back and explaining to him the results of the findings will be important. Asking him about diversion or misuse of stimulants might shed light on why he is asking for Dexedrine prescription. Using motivation interview technique to ask him to start seeing an addiction counselor will be an important step. Stimulant medications should not be prescribed to MM. It is very important that physicians do not become judgmental or condescending in these situations.

Literature Review Questions

Is the concept of feigning of mental illness new? Has it been recognized in the past?

The feigning of mental illness for external incentive has been recognized for centuries. In 1838, the Drs Beck & Beck noted, "Diseases are generally feigned from one of three causes—fear, shame, or hope of gain." They also noted that the most easily feigned illnesses are those with few to no physical manifestations or those based on self-report and in particular, "insanity, epilepsy, and pain."

What are the historical suggestions for detecting malingering using data from the book "Elements of Medical Jurisprudence" published in 1838 by Beck TR, Beck JB?

1. An external incentive is present.
2. No causative factor is present or the illness has a sudden onset.
3. The individual is resistant to receiving treatment.
4. Symptom complaints are inconsistent with the true illness.
5. The course of the disorder is inconsistent with the true illness.

Discuss the prevalence and epidemiology of malingering and ADHD?

Some researchers suggested that life-time prevalence rates of nonprescribed stimulants in college and university students range 5–43 % [1, 2].

As many as 50 % of students self-referred for an ADHD evaluation on campus were thought to have exaggerated their symptoms and performed on neuropsychological assessments in ways suggestive of malingering [3]. Similar findings were reported by [4]. Research on the feigning of ADHD outside of college populations is lacking; however, in one nationally representative study of adults, nearly 20 % of past-year nonmedical users indicated that they had obtained their medication fraudulently from a physician by misrepresenting their symptoms [5]. A recent study found that 10.5 % of female college students endorsed having ever used ADHD specific stimulant outside a doctor's prescription for the purpose of weight loss [6].

What are some of the reasons for malingering and faking ADHD symptoms?

- Obtain prescriptions for stimulant medications to enhance performance
- Gaining additional school services and accommodations (e.g., separate testing environments, longer testing times, reduced homework, and provision of a note taker)
- Use recreationally
- Sell as a Street Drug
  In general, money is not the only incentive for malingering in disability evaluations [7].

What are some of the common strategies used to fake ADHD?

Some authors [8] suggested that the following strategies have been used to fake ADHD symptoms:

- ADHD simulators reported that they tried to show difficulty paying attention and attempted to appear less intelligent.
- Slowly completing tasks.
- Trying to act like an acquaintance with ADHD.
- "Zoning out" or attending to distracting noises.
- Choosing incorrect answers, particularly on harder items.
- Skipping items.
- Responding quickly and carelessly while completing tasks.
- Being inattentive to verbal instructions or disobeying instructions.
- Selecting items on the Scale that matched DSM-IV criteria.
- Unfocusing their eyes or only focusing on the middle of the page (9 %).

- Beginning tasks before being told to begin.
- Pretending to have trouble remembering things.
- Acting confused or nervous.

Would self-report rating measures detect feigned ADHD?

Some authors indicated that self-report rating measures are not sensitive enough to allow the detection of feigned ADHD [9]. They suggested that self-report rating measures are easily simulated by patients without ADHD. They concluded that no questionnaire has proved sufficiently robust against false positives [10].

Would validity indices embedded in broad, objective personality inventories such as Minnesota Multiphasic Personality Inventory (MMPI) detect simulated ADHD?

Studies of the MMPI-2 and MMPI-2-RF (Restructured form, [11]) suggest that the measures of infrequently endorsed items related to psychopathology, Fp, and Fp-r (Infrequent Psychopathology Responses) demonstrate a promise in detecting simulated ADHD.

It appears that embedded indices of the MMPI-2 and MMPI-2-RF demonstrate more promise than do self-report ADHD questionnaires [10].

Give examples of neuropsychological tests

- Test of Variables of Attention (*TOVA*; Greenberg et al. 1996)
- Integrated Visual and Auditory Continuous Performance Test (*IVA CPT*)
- Woodcock–Johnson Psychoeducational Battery (Woodcock et al. 2001)
- Conners' Continuous Performance Test (*C-CPT*; Conners 1995)
- Trail Making Test Parts A and B [12]
- Wechsler Adult Intelligence Scale
- Neuropsychological Assessment Battery Numbers and Letters Test part A (NAB-NLA; White and Stern 2003)

What are some of the literature findings on the validity of using neuropsychological tests to detect ADHD simulators?

ADHD simulators are able to produce cognitive profiles that are relatively similar to individuals with ADHD. Earlier research suggested that the most promising neuropsychological tests appear to be Continuous performance tests (CPTs) [13–15] and the Stroop test [4, 16]. Other researchers noted that "*data are mixed*" [4, 13, 17].

Sollman et al. [16] reported that the C-CPT was not useful at discriminating individuals with ADHD from controls but possibly the different conclusions may reflect the nature of the samples used or small sample sizes.

Some authors found inconsistent results on CPT measures, with limitations to both sensitivity and specificity noted for both child and adult ADHD assessment. They mentioned that it is important to consider other disorders that can impact CPT performance prior to interpreting CPT impairment as indicative of ADHD. The authors encourage use of multiple measures during clinical evaluations of noncredible responses, in addition to considering evidence for external motivations for behaving noncredibly, before concluding that someone is malingering [4].

It is concluded that neuropsychological test data alone are insufficient and studies that use data from credible and noncredible patients highlight the necessity of effort assessment during ADHD evaluations [4, 17]. It is recommended to collect data from multiple sources for determination of ADHD [13].

Define Symptom Validity Tests (SVTs)?

Symptom validity testing (SVT) is an aspect of neuropsychological testing where separate scales, either embedded in neuropsychological test batteries, or included as additional elements, are used to establish the probability that a given test performance is affected by a tendency to fake bad, fake good, or malingering

Give examples of SVTS?

- Test of Memory Malingering (TOMM)
- Rey 15-Item Test
- Recognition Memory Test (RMT)
- Word Memory Test (WMT)
- Validity Indicator Profile (VIP)
- Computerized Assessment of Response Bias
- Portland Digit Recognition Test (PDRT)
- Victoria Symptom Validity Test (VSVT)
- Digit Memory Test (DMT)

What are some of the literature findings on the validity of using SVTs to detect ADHD simulators?

It appears that the most promising means of detecting malingered ADHD are SVTs that were originally designed to detect malingered cognitive symptoms. They are described as having excellent specificity, but inadequate sensitivity. However, combining SVTs may drastically increase the ability to identify malingerers [18].

The Word Memory Test (WMT) has been investigated and demonstrated some utility in detecting malingered ADHD [13, 17]. The WMT has been used to classify individuals as having poor effort in a number of studies [4, 17, 19, 20].

Victoria Symptom validity Test (VSVT) has also been used to identify some cases of malingering.

The final conclusion states that the ability to diagnose simulated ADHD drastically increases when three or more SVTs are failed [16, 17].

What are some of the clinical factors that may suggest malingering in ADHD assessment?

1. Marked inconsistencies, contradictions in reporting of symptoms.

   Example: Patient reported inability to read books because of inability to sustain attentions, but during the past month patient was able to read five different books and enjoys reading for hours even if the topic is not interesting.

2. Marked inconsistencies, contradictions between reported and observed symptoms.

   Example: Reported symptoms: patient reports being very hyperactive and always fidgeting with hands and feet, cannot sit in his place for more than half an hour.

   Observed symptoms: During a 2 h assessment, you did not observe any restlessness, hyperactivity, or inability to remain in seat.

3. Marked inconsistencies, contradictions between reported and observed level of function.

Example: Reported level of functioning: poor function in university but the records show A+ and GPA average of 4.2 each year.

4. Marked inconsistencies, contradictions between reported symptoms and psychological test results.

Example of reported symptoms: I was diagnosed with ADHD in grade 4 in school.

Observed: Obtaining the educational psychological assessment in school shows that patient was not diagnosed with ADHD.

5. Patient endorses improbable ADHD symptoms.

Examples: "I forget where I live all the time and has to ask for directions how to go home."

"I can never remember what year it is. My memory is really bad."

6. Patient is behaving in an unusual way during the interview: extremely guarded, uncooperative, hostile, evasive, responding with I do not know to simple questions.

What are some of the clinical tips that may guard against misdiagnosis in cases of malingered ADHD?

1. Consider the possibility of malingering and add to your differential diagnosis when indicated (see above factors).
2. Always do a complete assessment including:
   (a) Interview of parent or significant other and obtain collateral information as much as possible from different sources
   (b) Review of past educational records
   (c) Review of past medication – medical records
   (d) Get all past psychiatric/psychological records
   (e) Speak directly with the referring doctor if you are specialist
   (f) Ask about trouble with the law and any forensic history
   (g) Ask about secondary gains
3. Do not be rushed into filling out disability forms or other forms. ADHD is a chronic, lifetime illness – better to spend more time completing your assessment than reaching an inaccurate conclusion.
4. Do not be rushed or pressured into prescribing stimulant medications when patients have an agenda and insist on having a prescription without proper assessment.

References

1. Advokat C, Guidry D, Martino L (2008) Licit and illicit use of medications for Attention-Deficit Hyperactivity Disorder in undergraduate college students. J Am Coll Health 56(6):601–606
2. Kaye S, Darke S (2012) The diversion and misuse of pharmaceutical stimulants: what do we know and why should we care? Addiction 107(3):467–77. doi:10.1111/j.1360-0443.2011.03720.x, Review. PubMed PMID: 22313101

3. Sullivan BK, May K, Galbally L (2007) Symptom exaggeration by college adults in attention-deficit hyperactivity disorder and learning disorder assessments. Appl Neuropsychol 14:189–207

4. Suhr JA, Sullivan BK, Rodriguez JL (2011) The relationship of noncredible performance to continuous performance test scores in adults referred for attention-deficit/hyperactivity disorder evaluation. Arch Clin Neuropsychol 26(1):1–7

5. Novak SP, Kroutil LA, Williams RL, Van Brunt DL (2007) The nonmedical use of prescription ADHD medications: results from a national Internet panel. Subst Abus Treat Prev Policy 2:32

6. Gibbs EL, Kass AE, Eichen DM, Fitzsimmons-Craft EE, Trockel M, Wilfley DE (2016) Attention-deficit/hyperactivity disorder-specific stimulant misuse, mood, anxiety, and stress in college-age women at high risk for or with eating disorders. J Am Coll Health 64(4):300–8. doi:10.1080/07448481.2016.1138477, Epub 2016 Jan 29. PubMed PMID: 26822019; PubMed Central PMCID: PMC4904716

7. Clemow DB, Walker DJ (2014) The potential for misuse and abuse of medications in ADHD: a review. Postgrad Med 126(5):64–81

8. Frazier TW, Frazier AR, Busch RM, Kerwood MA, Demaree HA (2008) Detection of simulated ADHD and reading disorder using symptom validity measures. Arch Clin Neuropsychol 23:501–509

9. Tucha L, Sontag TA, Walitza S, Lange KW (2009) Detection of malingered attention deficit hyperactivity disorder. Atten Defic Hyperact Disord 1(1):47–53

10. Musso MW, Gouvier WD (2014) "Why is this so hard?" A review of detection of malingered ADHD in college students. J Atten Disord 18(3):186–201

11. Harp JP, Jasinski LJ, Shandera-Ochsner AL, Mason LH, Berry DTR (2011) Detection of malingered ADHD using the MMPI-2-RF. Psychol Inj Law 4:32–43

12. Reitan RM (1955) The relation of the trail making test to organic brain damage. J Consult Psychol 19(5):393–394

13. Lee Booksh R, Pella RD, Singh AN, Drew GW (2010) Ability of college students to simulate ADHD on objective measures of attention. J Atten Disord 13(4):325–338

14. Quinn CA (2003) Detection of malingering in assessment of adult ADHD. Arch Clin Neuropsychol 18:379–395

15. Leark RA, Dixon D, Hoffman T, Huynh D (2002) Fake bad test response bias on the test of variables of attention. Arch Clin Neuropsychol 17:335–342

16. Sollman MJ, Ranseen JD, Berry DT (2010) Detection of feigned ADHD in college students. Psychol Assess 22(2):325–335

17. Marshall P, Schroeder R, O'Brien J, Fischer R, Ries A, Blesi B et al (2010) Effectiveness of symptom validity measures in identifying cognitive and behavioral symptom exaggeration in adult attention deficit/hyperactivity disorder. Clin Neuropsychol 24:1204–1237

18. Jasinski LJ, Harp JP, Berry DT, Shandera-Ochsner AL, Mason LH, Ranseen JD (2011) Using symptom validity tests to detect malingered ADHD in college students. Clin Neuropsychol 25(8):1415–1428

19. Harrison AG, Rosenblum Y, Currie S (2010) Examining unusual digit span performance in a population of postsecondary students assessed for academic difficulties. Assessment 17(3):283–293

20. Harrison AG, Edwards MJ, Parker KCH (2007) Identifying students faking ADHD: preliminary findings and strategies for detection. Arch Clin Neuropsychol 22:577–588

Bibliography

Beck TR, Beck JB (1838) Elements of medical jurisprudence. Thomas Cowperthwait & Co., Philadelphia

Erdodi LA, Roth RM, Kirsch NL, Lajiness-O'neill R, Medoff B (2014) Aggregating validity indicators embedded in Conners' CPT-II outperforms individual cutoffs at separating valid from invalid performance in adults with traumatic brain injury. Arch Clin Neuropsychol 29(5):456–466

Fuermaier AB, Tucha L, Koerts J, Mueller AK, Lange KW, Tucha O (2012) Measurement of stigmatization towards adults with attention deficit hyperactivity disorder. PLoS One 7(12):e51755

Fuermaier AB, Tucha L, Mueller AK, Koerts J, Hauser J, Lange KW, Tucha O (2014) Stigmatization in teachers towards adults with attention deficit hyperactivity disorder. Springerplus 3:26

Hartung CM, Lefler EK, Canu WH, Stevens AE, Jaconis M, LaCount PA, Shelton CR, Leopold DR, Willcutt EG (2016) DSM-5 and other symptom thresholds for ADHD: which is the best predictor of impairment in college students? J Atten Disord. pii: 1087054716629216. [Epub ahead of print] PubMed PMID: 26903353

Hunt MG, Bienstock SW, Qiang JK (2012) Effects of diurnal variation on the Test of Variables of Attention performance in young adults with attention-deficit/hyperactivity disorder. Psychol Assess 24(1):166–172

Lefler EK, Sacchetti GM, Del Carlo DI (2016) ADHD in college: a qualitative analysis. Atten Defic Hyperact Disord. [Epub ahead of print] PubMed PMID: 26825556

Leopold DR, Willcutt EG (2016) DSM-5 and other symptom thresholds for ADHD: which is the best predictor of impairment in college students? J Atten Disord. pii: 1087054716629216

Loughan AR, Perna R (2014) Performance and specificity rates in the Test of Memory Malingering: an investigation into pediatric clinical populations. Appl Neuropsychol Child 3(1):26–30

Musso MW, Hill BD, Barker AA, Pella RD, Gouvier WD (2014) Utility of the personality assessment inventory for detecting malingered ADHD in college students. J Atten Disord. pii: 1087054714548031

Perugi G, Vannucchi G (2015) The use of stimulants and atomoxetine in adults with comorbid ADHD and bipolar disorder. Expert Opin Pharmacother 16(14):2193–2204

Rabiner DL (2013) Stimulant prescription cautions: addressing misuse, diversion and malingering. Curr Psychiatry Rep 15(7):375

Rios J, Morey LC (2013) Detecting feigned ADHD in later adolescence: an examination of three PAI-A negative distortion indicators. J Pers Assess 95(6):594–599

Schneider HE, Kirk JW, Mahone EM (2014) Utility of the test of memory malingering (TOMM) in children ages 4–7 years with and without ADHD. Clin Neuropsychol 28(7):1133–1145

Williamson KD, Combs HL, Berry DT, Harp JP, Mason LH, Edmundson M (2014) Discriminating among ADHD alone, ADHD with a comorbid psychological disorder, and feigned ADHD in a college sample. Clin Neuropsychol 28(7):1182–1196

Young JC, Gross AM (2011) Detection of response bias and noncredible performance in adult attention-deficit/hyperactivity disorder. Arch Clin Neuropsychol 26(3):165–175

ADHD and Obesity

3

Objectives
1. Understand the relationship between ADHD and obesity
2. List some of the different hypothesis that may explain the association between ADHD and obesity
3. Recognize the clinical and public health implications for the association between ADHD and obesity
4. Review some of the principals of management of patients with ADHD and obesity

3.1   The Case of Olga Oland

Patient Identification   Olga Oland is a 34-year-old female who lives in Halifax with her boyfriend and currently works at a local post office. She has two boys ages 11 and 8. She has been married to her husband for 14 years.

Circumstances of the Assessment   Olga made an appointment with you because she wants to go back to college and thinks she may have ADHD. Her older son was diagnosed last year and he is now successfully treated and doing much better in class.

Current Stressors   Olga mentioned that her relationship with her husband has been deteriorating for the past 2 years. She feels that he is not interested in spending any time with her and he finds every opportunity to stay outside the home and put more hours at work. She has been trying to lose some weight but her efforts were not successful. Her current weight is 224 Lbs with a BMI of 34 and she feels that her weight is contributing to her marital problems. Her younger son has several health problems that contributed to her stress. The post office has been very busy lately and the number of carless mistakes she made led her to receive a letter of warning from her employer.

© Springer International Publishing Switzerland 2017
J. Sadek, *Clinician's Guide to Adult ADHD Comorbidities*,
DOI 10.1007/978-3-319-39794-8_3

History of Present Illness Patient said since the diagnosis of her older son with ADHD, she started recognizing that she has similar symptoms for most of her life. She often cannot pay attention to details, cannot remember her appointments and must use a BlackBerry as a reminder system. She fidgets a lot, is described by others as a day dreamer, and as not a good listener. She used to leave her seat in class and later during long meetings. She feels embarrassed that others criticized her for butting into conversation. She frequently interrupts others and has difficulty organizing her work and her room. She described her car as a mess. One of the reasons she received a warning letter from her employer is because of the number of careless mistakes she makes. She also started several projects but never finished them including knitting gloves for her kids but not finishing them. She also mentioned the wall in her son's room that she started painting a year ago but never finished. She says her ability to sustain attention when reading is usually 5 min, then she drops the book and goes to do something else. She reported long-standing feelings of inner restlessness and feels that most of her symptoms started in primary school. The symptoms continued but she has never done anything about them. When she completed rating scales in the office, she missed several items on the scales.

Olga complains that her sleep is terrible, she has been feeling tired lately but she reported good mood, enjoyment of being around her kids on weekends. She never had suicidal thoughts. She eats a lot and described herself as an emotional eater. She started many diets but never followed through. She eats when frustrated or nervous and has no regular schedule for meals. She joined exercise classes but she got bored and stopped going. She eats lots of fast food and describes herself as impulsive eater.

She does not use street drugs and drinks a glass of wine with dinner on weekends.

No history of panic episodes and screening for GAD, OCD, phobia, PTSD, and social anxiety was unrevealing.

No past psychiatric evaluation.

Medical History No known allergies. Her cholesterol has been high but her blood pressure has been stable at 124/80. She had a concussion at age 14 during a car accident. Her children were both born by cesarean section.

Family History Olga has a 26-year-old sister. Her parents live together. Mom has an anxiety disorder and is treated with paroxetine 40 mg daily. She thinks her father has the same problems with inattention but he was never diagnosed.

Personal History Olga had an uncomplicated birth and development. She had no delay reaching her milestones.

During her primary school, she had numerous comments from teachers that she is day dreaming and not paying attention in class. She failed grade 7 and quit school after grade 11 to start low paying jobs. She returned to school 2 years later and obtained her high school diploma. She was bullied in school because of her obesity and she always feels insecure and inferior to others.

No reported problems with the law except for several traffic violations. Her parents were not well off but her needs were met.

She has been working at the post office for 7 years and gets along well with her coworkers. She said she always made lots of mistakes at work but her coworkers would help her and cover them up. Now that she has a new manager, her mistakes must be corrected or she will lose her job. She was fired once from work as a front store supervisor because she was frequently coming late to work and would not prepare the required weekly reports.

- Patient gave consent to talk to her family. Her mother reported the following problems from childhood to adulthood: getting bored easily, constant fidgeting, poor self-control and over eating, poor organizational skills (home, office, desk, or car is extremely messy and cluttered), trouble starting and finishing projects, frequently forgetting appointments, commitments, and deadlines, constantly losing or misplacing things (school books, home key), difficulty paying attention at home and at school and hated going to school.

3.2 Case Continued

After confirming her diagnosis of ADHD and obesity and completing her medical work up and obtaining collateral information, patient was prescribed melatonin 5 mg that improved her sleep. She was also prescribed a stimulant medication Adderall 10 mg (mixed amphetamine salts) AM that helped her ADHD symptoms and poor meal planning. She was able to follow a diet for 6 months and lost 20 Lbs. Olga also joined an education group about healthy eating and life style. She started learning more techniques on coping with ADHD from her psychologist and found psychosocial treatment helpful.

Literature Review Questions
Is there a relationship between ADHD and obesity?
Recent meta-analysis found statistically significant association between ADHD and obesity/overweight regardless of possible confounders. The pooled prevalence of obesity was increased by about 70 % in adults with ADHD and 40 % in children with ADHD compared with subjects without ADHD. The review also showed that gender did not significantly affect the association between ADHD and obesity [1]. Researchers support the link between ADHD symptoms and obesity. A model incorporating genetic, behavioral, and psychological factor was suggested to fit this association and concludes that individuals who have more ADHD symptoms and carry a genetic profile associated with greater DA activation in the brain reward areas appear more likely to overeat and, as a result, may be at increased risk of obesity. That recent research supports the "reward surfeit" view of obesity and challenges the hypothesis that diminished DA levels account for ADHD symptom–adiposity association [2].

What are some of the different hypothesis that may explain the association between ADHD and obesity?

Researchers suggested that several possibilities arise [1]. The first hypothesis is that ADHD could increase the risk of obesity particularly with the impulsive and inattentive components of ADHD. Expression of impulsivity with poor inhibitory control could reinforce abnormal eating behaviors that, in turn, would increase the likelihood of obesity. Inattention and poor planning might cause difficulties in adhering to regular eating patterns and dietary regimens. It may also be associated with lack of awareness of food intake.

The hyperactive component of ADHD might not decrease the risk of obesity since it might not be a constant but rather modulated by the context. For example, energy expenditure decreases while watching television, and children with ADHD have been shown to watch more television and engage in less physical activity than comparison subjects without ADHD. In addition, hyperactivity linked to restless behaviors may also include abnormal eating patterns. The true effect of ADHD subtypes, ADHD symptom severity or frequency, and other variables (e.g., watching television, sedentary activity) related to ADHD and obesity cannot be confirmed because of the paucity of data.

The second hypothesis is that ADHD and obesity share common biological risk factors, including genetic variants. ADHD and obesity may share dopaminergic dysfunctions underpinning reward deficiency processing, but this understanding needs to be better evaluated. Interestingly, a "reward deficiency syndrome," characterized by insufficient dopamine-related natural reinforcement that leads to "unnatural" immediate rewards (such as inappropriate eating), has been reported in both ADHD and obesity. In addition, oxidative stress, which is linked to obesity, has also been associated with ADHD.

The third hypothesis is that obesity or factors associated with it cause or mimic ADHD. For example sleep-disordered breathing and shorter or later sleep have been reported to manifest with ADHD-like symptoms

What are the clinical and public health implications for the association between ADHD and obesity?

The obesity associated with ADHD might explain why patients with ADHD are at increased risk for higher cholesterol levels and higher blood pressure. It is suggested that assessing the risk for obesity should be part of the assessment and management of ADHD. Clinicians should also screen for ADHD in individuals who are referred for obesity, especially those with a previous history of unsuccessful weight-loss attempts. Despite the high rate of comorbidity between depression or anxiety and obesity, its association with ADHD might be particularly significant for its potential treatment implications [1].

What is the impact of ADHD on weight loss effort?

Compared to patients without ADHD, patients with ADHD had five times the number of previous weight loss attempts, more emotional eating, double the fast food consumption, and 31 % who were able to lose 5 % of their body weight compared to 61 % in patients without ADHD [3].

What are the principals of management of patients with ADHD and obesity?

Complete assessment of all ADHD comorbid disorders such as depression, anxiety, sleep disorders, binge eating, obesity, and risk factors to determine the best order of treatment.

Multimodal treatment of ADHD should include psychosocial treatment and pharmacotherapy. Psychosocial treatment should also include psychoeducation on the interrelatedness of poor eating habits, late and short sleep, skipping meals, binge eating, and obesity. The ADHD symptoms of forgetfulness, poor planning, and impulsivity add to the complexity and longer duration of these behaviors. A patient's understanding of the relationship between factors may facilitate compliance for each step of treatment.

Treatment of comorbidity consists of treatment of the most severe disorder first, usually the mood disorder, with antidepressant such as selective serotonin reuptake inhibitor (SSRI) or other treatments. Melatonin may be added for the delayed sleep phase disorder to help reset the biological clock and lead to an earlier sleep onset and thus longer sleep duration. Sufficient sleep may improve mood and reduce carbohydrate craving, as well as the severity of ADHD symptoms.

Stimulant medications are usually recommended as the first line of line treatment [4]. Pharmacological treatment for ADHD cannot be proven to decrease the risk of obesity associated with ADHD based on correlational studies. Overall, there is limited empirical evidence on the short- and long-term effects of psychostimulants on weight [1]. The improved planning of meals and the ability to keep to a diet seem to be the most important contributions of the stimulant treatment for weight loss. Weight loss as a side effect of stimulants is usually limited and not long lasting [5]. ADHD treatment could also facilitate weight loss by improved self-directedness, improving day time energy, decreasing novelty seeking, and ability to pay attention to signals of hunger and satiety [6].

References

1. Cortese S, Moreira-Maia CR, St Fleur D, Morcillo-Peñalver C, Rohde LA, Faraone SV (2016) Association Between ADHD and Obesity: A Systematic Review and Meta-Analysis. Am J Psychiatry 173(1):34–43
2. Patte KA, Davis CA, Levitan RD, Kaplan AS, Carter-Major J, Kennedy JL (2016) A behavioral genetic model of the mechanisms underlying the link between obesity and symptoms of ADHD. J Atten Disord pii: 1087054715618793
3. CADDRA 2015. WWW.CADDRA.CA.
4. Pagoto SL, Curtin C, Bandini LG, Anderson SE, Schneider KL, Bodenlos JS, Ma Y (2010) Weight loss following a clinic-based weight loss program among adults with attention deficit/ hyperactivity disorder symptoms. Eat Weight Disord 15(3):e166-72.
5. Kooij JJ (2016) ADHD and obesity. Am J Psychiatry 173(1):1–2
6. Levy LD, Fleming JP, Klar D (2009) Treatment of refractory obesity in severely obese adults following management of newly diagnosed attention deficit hyperactivity disorder. Int J Obes (Lond) 33(3):326–34.

Bibliography

Aguirre Castaneda RL, Kumar S, Voigt RG, Leibson CL, Barbaresi WJ, Weaver AL, Killian JM, Katusic SK (2016) Childhood attention-deficit/hyperactivity disorder, sex, and obesity: a longitudinal population-based study. Mayo Clin Proc 91(3):352–361

Cortese S, Angriman M (2014) Attention-deficit/hyperactivity disorder, iron deficiency, and obesity: is there a link? Postgrad Med 126(4):155–170

Cortese S, Castellanos FX (2014) The relationship between ADHD and obesity: implications for therapy. Expert Rev Neurother 14(5):473–479

Fernell E, Landgren M (2014) Links between attention-deficit/hyperactivity disorder and obesity. Acta Paediatr 103(8):e328

Kummer A, Barbosa IG, Rodrigues DH, Rocha NP, Rafael Mda S, Pfeilsticker L, Silva AC, Teixeira AL (2016) Frequency of overweight and obesity in children and adolescents with autism and attention deficit/hyperactivity disorder. Rev Paul Pediatr 34(1):71–77

Lundahl A, Nelson TD (2014) Attention deficit hyperactivity disorder symptomatology and pediatric obesity: psychopathology or sleep deprivation? J Health Psychol

Nigg JT, Johnstone JM, Musser ED, Long HG, Willoughby MT, Shannon J (2016) Attention-deficit/hyperactivity disorder (ADHD) and being overweight/obesity: new data and meta-analysis. Clin Psychol Rev 43:67–79

Racicka E, Hanć T, Giertuga K, Bryńska A, Wolańczyk T (2015) Prevalence of overweight and obesity in children and adolescents with ADHD: the significance of comorbidities and pharmacotherapy. J Atten Disord

Reinblatt SP (2015) Are eating disorders related to attention deficit/hyperactivity disorder? Curr Treat Options Psychiatry 2(4):402–412

Reinblatt SP, Leoutsakos JM, Mahone EM, Forrester S, Wilcox HC, Riddle MA (2015) Association between binge eating and attention-deficit/hyperactivity disorder in two pediatric community mental health clinics. Int J Eat Disord 48(5):505–511

Schoenfelder EN, Kollins SH (2016) Topical Review: ADHD and Health-Risk Behaviors: Toward Prevention and Health Promotion. J Pediatr Psychol. 41(7):735-40. doi: 10.1093/jpepsy/jsv162

Seymour KE, Reinblatt SP, Benson L, Carnell S (2015) Overlapping neurobehavioral circuits in ADHD, obesity, and binge eating: evidence from neuroimaging research. CNS Spectr 20(4):401–411

Vitelli O, Miano S, Villa MP (2016) Response to the letter "What is the role of ADHD symptoms in obesity affecting cognitive outcome?". Sleep Med 17:164. doi:10.1016/j.sleep.2015.06.010

Yang R, Gao W, Li R, Zhao Z (2016) What is the role of ADHD symptoms in obesity affecting cognitive outcomes? Sleep Med 17:163. doi:10.1016/j.sleep.2015.06.013

ADHD Comorbidities with Depression, Anxiety, and Suicide

4

Objective

1. Describe some of the epidemiological data on ADHD and suicide
2. Understand the comorbidity rates of ADHD and depression
3. Describe the link between ADHD and suicide
4. Review the relationship between ADHD medication and suicide
5. Review some possible explanations of the increased suicide risk in patients with ADHD
6. List some of the suicide risk assessment tools
7. Describe the management approaches for management of ADHD patients with depression or suicidality

4.1 The Case of David Dunn

Identification DD is a 41-year-old man who lives alone in a house in a small town in Nova Scotia. He works as an independent lawyer and has his own office. He has been recently divorced.

Chief Complaint Patient referred himself to the emergency room complaining of depression.

Stressors:

1. He received his final divorce papers 3 months ago. He called his ex-wife 8 days ago to tell her that they should get back together and she called the police and warned him not to contact her again.
2. He has been in a serious financial difficulty after the divorce.
3. Lately he has been unable to go to his office and the clients had been calling him looking to transfer their files away.

© Springer International Publishing Switzerland 2017
J. Sadek, *Clinician's Guide to Adult ADHD Comorbidities*,
DOI 10.1007/978-3-319-39794-8_4

History of Present Illness Patient said that he has been feeling depressed for the past 6 months. His mood is low and irritable. He lost 18 Lbs and has no appetite. His energy is poor and he cannot sleep at night until 2 or 3 AM. He feels guilty and responsible for the divorce because he was not paying attention to his wife. He enjoys golfing and playing tennis but he has not done any activity for 6 months. His concentration has been poor and feels that his memory is deteriorating. He stopped talking to his family and is not interested in reaching out to his friends. He was asked if he had thoughts of ending his life. He said "Only this week. I wish I could end it all." He had some thoughts of hanging himself but he would not do it because of his elderly parents. He had no previous suicide attempts and this was his first time to consider suicide. No active symptoms of mania and he never had manic episodes in the past.

Alcohol and substance use screening: Patient said he drinks a bottle of wine on weekends and never used street drugs. He is not a smoker.

Anxiety Screening DD is very worried about his life without his partner. He is also worried about his finances, his work, his elderly parents, and his health. He feels irritable and tense. He frequently feels restless and on the edge. Before bedtime, all the anxious thoughts come to his mind and prevent him from sleeping. He is unable to control his anxiety and feels that he is no longer able to function. Screening for phobia, PTSD, OCD, and panic disorder was unrevealing.

Psychosis Screening Denied hallucinatory experience. He has no delusions. His behavior and speech are organized and his thought process is clear and organized.

Past Psychiatric History He said his only encounter with mental health was at age 10 when he was seen by a psychiatrist because of problems with anxiety and paying attention in class. He thinks he was diagnosed with anxiety and was seen several times by a psychologist.

Medical History Patient has no known drug allergies. He has acid reflux and was prescribed omeprazole 20 mg daily. He had an appendectomy at age 16 but otherwise he is healthy.

Family History Patient has one younger brother with ADHD. His parents have been married for many years. Mother had depression and was treated with Citalopram. Father started having problems with short term memory. He was a successful businessman.

Personal and Social History Patient was born in Halifax, NS, Canada. He said he is not aware of any problems in his mother's pregnancy. His delivery was complicated by a cord around his neck. He had some speech delay.

He said his parents were very loving and caring but he had great difficulty separating from them and would refuse to go to school so he would not separate from his mother. When his father would come late from work, he would cry and feel that something bad might have happened to him. He had many friends as a child but now he has only 3 of them. He had three girl friends before his wife that left and divorced him. He felt that he can no longer have any other partners.

DD was a good student except for mathematics. He never failed any grades but failed math classes in grade 9 and 11. His parents were able to have a private tutor for him during high school and his mother spent a lot of time helping him finish his homework every day after school. He enjoyed playing sports and was part of the school badminton team. Teachers liked him because he was shy and quiet but he was always reminded to finish his homework and stop day dreaming in class. He had problems with organization and was asked to keep his desk clean and tidy. He was asked frequently to stay after hours to finish his work. His father wanted him to go to law school and he worked very hard to get there and graduate. He failed several courses in university and was placed on academic probation. He graduated from law school and spent 1 year articling then joined a small firm but the deadlines were very hard to meet so he started his own firm. He is easily distracted by sound and movements so he keeps many signs in the office to keep quiet. To keep his appointments organized, he hired two secretaries to look after organizing his day and reminding him with appointments. He requires frequent text messages and phone calls to keep him organized. He also has a legal assistant to help him with the details of the cases. He often avoids complex business cases that require sustained attention.

DD started crying describing his difficulties. He said he started his career 6 years ago and he was very supported by his partner, and once she left his life started falling apart.

Diagnostic Considerations and Plan:

First consideration is to the patient's suicidal thoughts. Patient has several risk factors for suicide including recent crisis, recent loss, major depressive episode, anhedonia, restlessness, and anxiety.

He has a plan to hang himself.

After discussing with the patient, he agreed to be admitted to a short stay inpatient unit to stay for few days for his own safety. He was started on escitalopram (Cipralex) 10 mg in the morning for major depressive episode and generalized anxiety disorder in addition to trazodone 50 mg at bedtime.

Complete physical examination and routine blood work were done in hospital and did not change the diagnostic impressions.

He agreed to have a family meeting with his parents who were quite pleased to offer support.

Patient's sleep improved and in 6 days he was no longer having suicidal thoughts. He agreed to stay with his parents after discharge and they were happy to support him.

He was seen weekly at the outpatient department and he continued to improve. In 8 weeks his depression resolved and his anxiety was much improved.

The collateral information from his parents confirmed that he has long standing symptoms of ADHD inattentive type. He agreed to start a stimulant medication while he was planning to return to work in 4 month after the admission. He was warned about the adverse effects of the stimulants including possible increase in anxiety. Patient tolerated the long acting methylphenidate 30 mg very well and he felt some improvement at his work performance. The dosage was increased to 40 mg then 50 mg 1 week later but at that dose his anxiety worsened so MPH was cut back from 50 to 40 mg. He tolerated the 40 mg well and continued to take his antidepressant and Trazodone.

Literature Review Questions
What are some of the findings of the epidemiological data on ADHD and suicide?

A recent large population based study in Sweden found that individuals with ADHD had an increased risk of both attempted and completed suicide compared with matched control participants (OR = 8.46 [95 % CI, 8.07–8.87] and OR = 12.22 [95 % CI, 8.67–17.22], respectively), even after adjusting for comorbid psychiatric disorders (OR = 3.62 [95 % CI, 3.29–3.98] and OR = 5.91 [95 % CI, 2.45–14.27], respectively [26]. In the UK, the rate of self-harm in 11–15-year-olds with hyperkinetic disorder was 8.5 % [14]; ADHD was found to occur more frequently in suicidal groups than control [22].

What are the comorbidity rates of ADHD and depression?

National Comorbidity Survey Replication study found that the prevalence rates of major depressive disorder (MDD) in adults with ADHD was 18.6 % (SE 4.2) and in adults without ADHD was 7.8 % (SE 0.4) with an odds ratio (OR) of 2.7 [25].

The prevalence rate of ADHD in patients with major depressive disorder was ranging from 5 to 16 % in several studies [6].

A common notion is that the cumulative effects of ADHD-related impairments and the negative environmental circumstances triggered by these may lead some youths with ADHD to eventually develop depression [16].

What is the relationship between ADHD and suicide?

ADHD is associated with an increased risk of both attempted and completed suicide.

While ADHD can be viewed as an independent risk factor for suicide, some authors suggest that the association between ADHD and suicide is rather to be mediated by the symptoms of comorbid disorders as mood or anxiety disorders [2].

Recent study suggested that ADHD symptoms were linked to suicidal behavior after controlling for comorbid conditions [40].

What are the possible explanations of the increased suicide risk in patients with ADHD?

1. *Comorbid disorders*:

   Some authors suggest reported significant associations between ADHD and several psychiatric disorders.

   ADHD patients compared to controls are more likely to have psychiatric comorbidity and more likely to attempt suicide. Examples of comorbid disorders with ADHD:

Alcohol, substance and nicotine use disorders

Mood disorders, major depressive disorder, bipolar disorder

Anxiety disorders, obsessive–compulsive disorder, posttraumatic stress disorder, and phobia

Somatoform disorder and sleep disorders [24, 30, 32]

    Comorbid depression and ADHD predisposed to more lethal suicide attempts and more desire to end their life [31] and associated with a higher rate of suicidal ideation and attempts [5, 34].

    Substance abuse, co-occurring with ADHD, is associated with an increased risk of suicide and suicide attempts [1, 20].

    Alcohol-dependent adults with ADHD showed higher risk of developing suicidal behavior than those without ADHD [10].

    Patients with antisocial personality disorder (ASPD) and comorbid ADHD have increased rate of self injurious behavior and suicide attempts [39].

2. *Cognitive impairment and personality traits*

    Impaired decision-making is a vulnerability in suicidal behavior [23] and ADHD [27, 29].

    Poor decision making can be a result of the impulsivity which is an important symptom of ADHD.

    One study suggested that the personality trait of impulsivity contributed to attempting suicide.

3. *Neurobiology*

    Lower cerebrospinal fluid concentration of the dopamine metabolite homovanillic acid (HVA) as well as of the serotonin metabolite 5-hydroxyindoleacetic acid (5-HIAA) [38] have been suggested to be a possible underlying mechanism in suicide and ADHD.

    A decreased level of dopamine in one of the components of the reward system, specifically the nucleus accumbens, was found to be low in the postmortem brains of depressed suicide patients and also in ADHD patients [7].

    A recent large population based study in Sweden suggested that there is an increased risk of both attempted and completed suicide in ADHD patients and their first degree relatives. The study suggested that shared genetic factors are important for this association and that individuals with ADHD and their family members are important targets for suicide prevention and treatment [26].

What are the correlates of having both ADHD and depression in adult population?

Some researchers found that ADHD patients may have earlier age of onset of depression, more depressive episodes, greater anxiety disorder comorbidity, greater substance abuse comorbidity, and greater antisocial personality disorder comorbidity or history of violence [28].

What are some of the challenges in diagnosis of ADHD in presence of depression or vice versa?

Symptom overlap between ADHD and MDD may lead to misdiagnosis. Some of the DSM V criteria for diagnosis of MDD might be associated with ADHD to some degree such as poor concentration, insomnia, psychomotor agitation, or retardation and fatigue. On the other hand, inattentive symptoms of ADHD such as distractibility, difficulty sustaining attention, or hyperactivity symptoms such as difficulty sitting still might mimic symptoms of depression. It is important to make the distinction between demoralization, an outgrowth of the negative consequences of ADHD, and a clinical diagnosis of major depression that is episodic [15].

What is the economic Impact of ADHD and Depression Comorbidity?

Presence of comorbid ADHD and depression resulted in marginal costs approximately 29–30% higher than the costs specifically attributed to depression alone [13].

What are the management approaches of ADHD and Depression?

Some evidence suggests that ADHD treatments may be less effective in patients with active depression and may lead to an exacerbation of dysphoria, poor sleep, and decreased appetite [41].

In patients with moderate to severe depression and ADHD, some clinical guidelines recommend to start by assessing for suicide risk and treating depression first [19].

In patients with mild depression and ADHD, the recommendations suggest to continue to assess for suicide risk, start ADHD treatment, and add an antidepressant when indicated [19].

In an open-label study, adults with ADHD in presence of depressive disorder were first treated with fluoxetine or sertraline for MDD followed by a stimulant for ADHD. The study concluded that this combination therapy was well tolerated and appeared to be effective in ameliorating both ADHD and depressive symptoms [12]. Some researchers suggested that antidepressants with noradrenergic and dopaminergic activity, particularly bupropion, may have some benefit in improving ADHD symptoms and depressive symptoms.

Selective serotonin reuptake inhibitors (SSRI) monotherapy was effective in treating depression but had limited benefit for ADHD symptoms.

Atomoxetine which is a noradrenergic reuptake inhibitor (NRI) demonstrates an efficacy for ADHD symptoms with a moderate effect size of 0.63 but limited results for treatment of depression [3].

For general treatment of depression, some authors suggested that sertraline or escitalopram should be considered first line for treatment of depression because of their efficacy, side effects profile, and cost. Bupropion is often a first-line alternative to sertraline, because of its lack of sexual side effects; although it has less efficacy for anxiety disorders, it is helpful for other comorbidities, such as tobacco dependence and ADHD. Both paroxetine and mirtazepine may often be less prescribed because of side effects of sedation and weight gain; however, these side effects may be advantageous for those whose depressive symptoms include insomnia and excessive weight loss [9].

Drug-drug interaction between ADHD medications and antidepressants should also be considered since methylphenidate (MPH) should not be used in patients receiving monoamine oxidase inhibitors (MAOI) due to a risk for hypertensive crisis or serotonin syndrome [11].

Since SSRIs are metabolized in the liver, while 80% of methylphenidate is metabolized extrahepatically, there has been little concern with this combination [18].

Cognitive behavioral therapy may be helpful in patients with depression and ADHD and often in conjunction with medications. Other psychosocial treatments for ADHD can also be employed such as organizational skills, anger management training, social skills, and education about the illness and the medication [21].

What is the relationship between ADHD medication and Suicide?

Atomoxetine
In 2005, both the United States Food and Drug Administration and Health Canada
  warned of increased rates of suicidal ideation among patients taking atomoxetine
  in placebo-controlled trials. The latter published meta-analysis that prompted the
  warnings after reviewing 12 studies comparing outcomes in children treated with
  atomoxetine or placebo. Suicidal ideation was reported to have occurred in 5
  (0.37 %) of 1357 children given atomoxetine, but in none of 851 children receiving placebo [4].
As a result, health providers were advised to closely monitor children and adolescents treated with atomoxetine for aggravation of symptoms such as agitation,
  irritability, suicidal thinking, or behaviors and unusual changes in behavior.
A case report was published in 2008 of acute agitation and suicidal ideation in an
  11-year-old boy after commencing atomoxetine [35].
Stimulant Medications
One study that examined the adult outcomes of childhood stimulant medication
  in a relatively small group of 32 subjects found that for 20 young adults, the
  childhood treatment had no lasting effect, but for 11 others the positive effects
  lasted long after treatment was discontinued. Higher dosage of medication
  was associated with fewer diagnoses of alcoholism and with fewer suicide
  attempts [33].
There are seven comparator trials of atomoxetine and methylphenidate, five of
  which were randomized double blind and included in the analysis of suicide risk
  while receiving ADHD medications. In total, there were five events using FDA
  coding 1–4, atomoxetine 3/559, and methylphenidate 2/465. All events using
  FDA coding 1–4 were suicidal ideation: there were no suicide attempts nor completed suicides and there was no difference in risk between atomexetine and
  methylphenidate with a Mantel-Haenszel risk ratio of 0.52 (95 % CI; 0.06, 4.54).
  Mantel-Haenszel risk ratio (MH) was used for categorical data replacing the
  odds ratio (OR) [8].

What Do I tell Patients and families when asked about suicide and ADHD medication?

Some patients may inquire about suicide risk when taking ADHD medications particularly in North America after Health Canada Announcement in March 2015: "ADHD drugs may increase risk of suicidal thoughts and behaviors in some people; benefits still outweigh risks".

Health Canada reported increased risk of suicidal ideation when the ADHD medication was started, when the dose was changed, and when the medication was stopped. Mood symptoms may be induced by psychostimulants (irritability, dysphoria).

It was suggested that while patients and their families should be made aware of the increased risk of suicidal thoughts and behaviors among people who have

ADHD, families should also be told this strong warning on ADHD medications should not be a cause for panic and that:

- Patients taking ADHD medications, as well as their parents, families, and friends should monitor for suicidal thoughts and behaviors.
- Patients and families be encouraged to report any distressing thoughts or feelings immediately to their doctor. This applies at all stages of treatment and even after ADHD therapy has been stopped.
- ADHD medication should not be changed or stopped without medical advice.
- Healthcare professionals monitor patients more closely around the start of treatment, at dose change, and when medication is stopped.
- Suicide risk assessment for patients at moderate or high risk of suicide is essential and a clear management plan should be developed [19].

Give examples of questions that can be asked to screen for suicide?

Example #1:
Sometimes people who get upset or feel bad wish they were dead or feel they'd be better off dead. Have you ever had these types of thoughts? When? Do you feel that way now? Was there ever another time you felt that way?

Example #2:
Do you feel that the past few weeks were very stressful and difficult that you wished you were dead? Did these thoughts start after you took the medication?

Are there tools that I can use in working with suicidal patients?
Several tools are available; however no specific tool has been designed for ADHD patients. None of the tools can predict suicide but would help the clinician during the assessment to cover the important areas before making a decision on the suicide risk level. Suicide risk assessment is mainly based on clinical judgment.

Examples:
Beck Scale for Suicide Ideation (BSS®), Beck Hopelessness Scale (BHS), Columbia-Suicide Severity Rating Scale (C-SSRS), Mental Health Environment of Care Checklist (MHECC), Nurses Global Assessment of Suicide Risk (NGASR), Reasons for Living Inventory (RFL), Scale for Impact of Suicidality – Management, Assessment and Planning of Care (SIS-MAP), Modified Scale for Suicide Ideation (SSI-M)

Sadek Assessment Tool of Suicidality (SATS): Full tool is included as appendix S Suicidal Behaviors Questionnaire (SBQ)

Suicide Intent Scale (SIS)
Suicide Probability Scale (SPS)
Tool for the Assessment of Suicide Risk (TASR)

More information on the above tools are found at the Suicide Risk Assessment Guide by the Ontario Hospital Association at https://www.oha.com/KnowledgeCentre/Documents

Give examples of tools that can be used in assessment of psychiatric comorbidity of ADHD?

Structured Clinical Interview (SCID–1/P)
First MB, Spitzer RL, Gibbon M, et al. Structured Clinical Interview for Axis I DSM-IV Disorders – Patient Edition (With Psychotic Screen) (SCID–1/P) (Version 2.0). *New York, NY: Biometrics Research, New York State Psychiatric Institute; 1996.*
Symptom Checklist–90 (SCL–90) Derogatis LR.
Symptom Checklist–90 (Revised): Administration, Scoring, and Procedures Manual II. Towson, MD: Clinical Psychometric Research; 1992.

How Should I Manage Suicidal Thoughts/Behavior During treatment with ADHD medications?

- Psychiatric history should be taken; this should routinely include an assessment of suicidality, either via general enquiry or via a standardized suicidality rating tool [37].
- Observe patients for the emergence of depression, irritability, and suicidal ideation as part of the routine monitoring. Determine whether the patient is expressing suicidal ideation, intent, plan, or is there a history of chronic self-harm behavior as in a personality disorder.
- Families and caregivers should be advised of the need to recognize any appearance of emotional change, self-injurious thinking, suicidal ideation, and irritability [17].
- Caution is required when prescribing ADHD drugs to patients with a past history of serious suicidal attempt or current untreated severe and impairing depression.
- In the case of ADHD and concurrent suicidal ideation in the context of a major depressive episode, the clinician should focus initially on the treatment of the disorder that is the most severe and impairing, i.e., the depressive disorder and its potentially life threatening complications (e.g., suicidality) [36].
- If suicidal ideation emerges during ADHD treatment, urgent psychiatric evaluation should be arranged.
- Consideration should be given to reducing the dose and/or other changes in the therapeutic regimen, including the possibility of discontinuing the medication, especially if these symptoms are severe or abrupt in onset, or were not part of the patient's presenting symptoms.
- It should, however, not automatically be assumed that any suicidal ideation or attempt is an adverse effect of medication [42].

References

1. Arias AJ et al (2008) Correlates of co-occurring ADHD in drugdependent subjects: prevalence and features of substance dependence and psychiatric disorders. Addict Behav 33(9): 1199–1207
2. Balazs J, Miklosi M, Kereszteny A, Dallos G, Gadoros J (2014) Attention-deficit hyperactivity disorder and suicidality in a treatment naïve sample of children and adolescents. J Affect Disord 152–154:282–287
3. Bangs ME, Emslie GJ, Spencer TJ et al; Atomoxetine ADHD and Comorbid MDD Study Group (2007) Efficacy and safety of atomoxetine in adolescents with attention-deficit/hyperactivity disorder and major depression. J Child Adolesc Psychopharmacol 17(4):407–20
4. Bangs ME et al (2008) Meta-analysis of suicide-related behavior events in patients treated with atomoxetine. J Am Acad Child Adolesc Psychiatry 47(2):209–218
5. Biederman J et al (2008) New insights into the comorbidity between ADHD and major depression in adolescent and young adult females. J Am Acad Child Adolesc Psychiatry 47(4):426–434
6. Bond DJ, Hadjipavlou G, Lam RW et al; Canadian Network for Mood and Anxiety Treatments (CANMAT) Task Force (2012) The Canadian Network for Mood and Anxiety Treatments (CANMAT) task force recommendations for the management of patients with mood disorders and comorbid attention-deficit/hyperactivity disorder. Ann Clin Psychiatry 24(1):23–37
7. Bowden C, Cheetham SC, Lowther S, Katona CL, Crompton MR, Horton RW (1997) Reduced dopamine turnover in the basal ganglia of depressed suicides. Brain Res 769(1):135–140
8. Bushe CJ, Savill NC (2013) Suicide related events and attention deficit hyperactivity disorder treatments in children and adolescents: a meta-analysis of atomoxetine and methylphenidate comparator clinical trials. Child Adolesc Psychiatr Ment Health 7:19
9. Carlat DA (2012) Evidence bsed somatic treatment of depression in adults. Psych Clin N Am 35:131–142
10. Cottencin O, Nandrino JL, Karila L, Mezerette C, Danel T (2009) A case-comparison study of executive functions in alcohol-dependent adults with maternal history of alcoholism. Eur Psychiatry 24(3):195–200
11. Evans C, Blackburn D, Butt P, Dattani D (2004) Use and abuse of methylphenidate in attention-deficit/hyperactivity disorder beware of legitimate prescriptions being diverted. Can Pharmacists J/Revue des Pharmaciens du Can 137(6):30–35
12. Findling RL (1996) Open-label treatment of comorbid depression and attentional disorders with co-administration of serotonin reuptake inhibitors and psychostimulants in children, adolescents, and adults: a case series. J Child Adolesc Psychopharmacol 6(3):165–175
13. Fishman PA, Stang PE, Hogue SL (2007) Impact of comorbid attention deficit disorder on the direct medical costs of treating adults with depression in managed care. J Clin Psychiatry 68(2):248–253
14. Furczyk K, Thome J (2014) Adult ADHD and suicide. Atten Defic Hyperact Disord 6(3):153–158
15. Goodman D, Happell B (2006) The efficacy of family intervention in adolescent mental health. Int J Psychiatr Nurs Res 12(1):1364–1377
16. Goodman DW, Thase ME (2009) Recognizing ADHD in adults with comorbid mood disorders: implications for identification and management. Postgrad Med 121(5):20–30
17. Graham J et al (2011) European guidelines on managing adverse effects of medication for ADHD. Eur Child Adolesc Psychiatry 20(1):17–37
18. Greenhill LL, Pliszka S, Dulcan MK et al; American Academy of Child and Adolescent Psychiatry (2002) Practice parameter for the use of stimulant medications in the treatment of children, adolescents, and adults. J Am Acad Child Adolesc Psychiatry 41(2 Suppl):26S–49S
19. Health Canada warning on ADHD medications: http://healthycanadians.gc.ca/recall-alert-rappel-avis/hc-sc/2015/52759a-eng.php
20. Huntley Z et al (2012) Rates of undiagnosed attention deficit hyperactivity disorder in London drug and alcohol detoxification units. BMC Psychiatry 6(12):223
21. Hyperlink: http://www.caddra.ca

22. Impey M, Heun R (2012) Completed suicide, ideation and attempt in attention deficit hyperactivity disorder. Acta Psychiatr Scand 125(2):93–102
23. Jollant F, Guillaume S, Jaussent I, Bellivier F, Leboyer M, Castelnau D, Malafosse A, Courtet P (2007) Psychiatric diagnoses and personality traits associated with disadvantageous decision-making. Eur Psychiatry 22(7):455–461, Epub 2007 Aug 30
24. Keresztény A, Dallos G, Miklósi M, Róka A, Gadoros J, Balazs J (2012) Comparing the comorbidity of attention-deficit/hyperactivity disorder in childhood and adolescence. Psychiatr Hung 27(3):165–173
25. Kessler RC, Adler L, Barkley R et al (2006) The prevalence and correlates of adult ADHD in the United States: results from the National Comorbidity Survey Replication. Am J Psychiatry 163(4):716–723
26. Ljung T, Chen Q, Lichtenstein P, Larsson H (2014) Common etiological factors of attention-deficit/hyperactivity disorder and suicidal behavior: a population-based study in Sweden. JAMA Psychiatry 71(8):958–964
27. Masunami T, Okazaki S, Maekawa H (2009) Decision-making patterns and sensitivity to reward and punishment in children with attention-deficit hyperactivity disorder. Int J Psychophysiol 72(3):283–288
28. McIntyre RS, Kennedy SH, Soczynska JK et al (2010) Attention-deficit/hyperactivity disorder in adults with bipolar disorder or major depressive disorder: results from the international mood disorders collaborative project. Prim Care Companion J Clin Psychiatry 12(3)
29. Miller M, Sheridan M, Cardoos SL, Hinshaw SP (2013) Impaired decision-making as a young adult outcome of girls diagnosed with attention-deficit/hyperactivity disorder in childhood. J Int Neuropsychol Soc 19(1):110–114
30. Murphy KR, Barkley RA, Bush T (2002) Young adults with attention deficit hyperactivity disorder: subtype differences in comorbidity, educational, and clinical history. J Nerv Ment Dis 190(3):147–157
31. Nasser EH, Overholser JC (1999) Assessing varying degrees of lethality in depressed adolescent suicide attempters. Acta Psychiatr Scand 99(6):423–431
32. Park S et al (2011) Prevalence, correlates, and comorbidities of adult ADHD symptoms in Korea: results of the Korean epidemiologic catchment area study. Psychiatry Res 186(2–3):378–383
33. Paternite CE, Loney J, Salisbury H, Whaley MA (1999) Childhood inattention-overactivity, aggression, and stimulant medication history as predictors of young adult outcomes. J Child Adolesc Psychopharmacol 9(3):169–184
34. Patros CH, Hudec KL, Alderson RM, Kasper LJ, Davidson C, Wingate LR (2013) Symptoms of attention-deficit/hyperactivity disorder (ADHD) moderate suicidal behaviors in college students with depressed mood. J Clin Psychol 69(9):980–993
35. Paxton GA, Cranswick NE (2008) Acute suicidality after commencing atomoxetine. J Paediatr Child Health 44(10):596–598
36. Pliszka SR, Crismon ML, Hughes CW, Corners CK, Emslie GJ, Jensen PS, McCracken JT, Swanson JM, Lopez M, Texas Consensus Conference Panel on Pharmacotherapy of Childhood Attention Deficit Hyperactivity Disorder (2006) The Texas Children's Medication Algorithm Project: revision of the algorithm for pharmacotherapy of attention-deficit/hyperactivity disorder. J Am Acad Child Adolesc Psychiatry 45(6):642–657
37. Posner MI, Rothbart MK (2007) Research on attention networks as a model for the integration of psychological science. Annu Rev Psychol 58:1–23
38. Rydén E, Thase ME, Stråht D, Aberg-Wistedt A, Bejerot S, Landén M (2009) A history of childhood attention-deficit hyperactivity disorder (ADHD) impacts clinical outcome in adult bipolar patients regardless of current ADHD. Acta Psychiatr Scand 120(3):239–246
39. Semiz UB et al (2008) Effects of diagnostic comorbidity and dimensional symptoms of attention-deficit-hyperactivity disorder in men with antisocial personality disorder. Aust N Z J Psychiatry 42(5):405–413
40. Stickley A, Koyanagi A, Ruchkin V, Kamio Y (2016) Attention-deficit/hyperactivity disorder symptoms and suicide ideation and attempts: findings from the adult psychiatric morbidity survey 2007. J Affect Disord 189:321–328

41. Weiss M, Hechtman L, Adult ADHD Research Group (2006) A randomized double-blind trial of paroxetine and/or dextroamphetamine and problem-focused therapy for attention-deficit/hyperactivity disorder in adults. J Clin Psychiatry 67(4):611–619
42. Young J (2008) Common comorbidities seen in adolescents with attention-deficit/hyperactivity disorder. Adolesc Med State Art Rev 19(2):216–228, vii, Review. PubMed PMID: 18822828

Bibliography

Asberg M, Traskman L, Thoren P (1976) 5-HIAA in the cerebrospinal fluid. A biochemical suicide predictor? Arch Gen Psychiatry 33(10):1193–1197

Barbaresi WJ et al (2013) Mortality, ADHD, and psychosocial adversity in adults with childhood ADHD: a prospective study. Pediatrics 131(4):637–644

Blum K et al (2008) Attention-deficit-hyperactivity disorder and reward deficiency syndrome. Neuropsychiatr Dis Treat 4(5):893–918

Chen Q, Sjölander A, Runeson B, D'Onofrio BM, Lichtenstein P, Larsson H (2014) Drug treatment for attention-deficit/hyperactivity disorder and suicidal behaviour: register based study. BMJ 348:g3769

Chronis-Tuscano A et al (2010) Very early predictors of adolescent depression and suicide attempts in children with attention-deficit/hyperactivity disorder. Arch Gen Psychiatry 67(10):1044–1051

Corruble E et al (2003) Defense styles, impulsivity and suicide attempts in major depression. Psychopathology 36(6):279–284

Do Mantyla T, Still J, Gullberg S, Del Missier F (2012) Decision making in adults with ADHD. J Atten Disord 16(2):164–173

Fayyad J et al (2007) Cross-national prevalence and correlates of adult attention-deficit hyperactivity disorder. Br J Psychiatry 190:402–409

Goldston DB et al (2009) Psychiatric diagnoses as contemporaneous risk factors for suicide attempts among adolescents and young adults: developmental changes. J Consult Clin Psychol 77(2):281–290

Goodman G, Gerstadt C, Pfeffer CR, Stroh M, Valdez A (2008) ADHD and aggression as correlates of suicidal behavior in assaultive prepubertal psychiatric inpatients. Suicide Life Threat Behav 38(1):46–59

Greening L et al (2008) Pathways to suicidal behaviors in childhood. Suicide Life Threat Behav 38(1):35–45

Gunter TD, Chibnall JT, Antoniak SK, McCormick B, Black DW (2012) Relative contributions of gender and traumatic life experience to the prediction of mental disorders in a sample of incarcerated offenders. Behav Sci Law 30(5):615–630

Hardy SE (2009) Methylphenidate for the treatment of depressive symptoms, including fatigue and apathy, in medically ill older adults and terminally ill adults. Am J Geriatr Pharmacother 7(1):34–59

Hinshaw SP (2012) Prospective follow-up of girls with attention-deficit/hyperactivity disorder into early adulthood: continuing impairment includes elevated risk for suicide attempts and self-injury. J Consult Clin Psychol 80(6):1041–1051

Hurtig T, Taanila A, Moilanen I, Nordstrom T, Ebeling H (2012) Suicidal and self-harm behaviour associated with adolescent attention deficit hyperactivity disorder-a study in the Northern Finland Birth Cohort 1986. Nord J Psychiatry 66:320–328

Klein-Schwartz W (2002) Abuse and toxicity of methylphenidate. Curr Opin Pediatr 14(2):219–223. Review

Kollins SH (2008) A qualitative review of issues arising in the use of psycho-stimulant medications in patients with ADHD and co-morbid substance use disorders. Curr Med Res Opin 24(5):1345–1357. doi:10.1185/030079908X280707, Epub 2008 Apr 1. Review. PubMed PMID: 18384709

Kollins SH (2008) ADHD, substance use disorders, and psychostimulant treatment: current literature and treatment guidelines. J Atten Disord 12(2):115–125. doi:10.1177/1087054707311654, Epub 2008 Jan 11. Review. PubMed PMID: 18192623

Manor I et al (2010) Possible association between attention deficit hyperactivity disorder and attempted suicide in adolescents – a pilot study. Eur Psychiatry 25(3):146–150

McCarthy S, Cranswick N, Potts L, Taylor E, Wong IC (2009) Mortality associated with attention-deficit hyperactivity disorder (ADHD) drug treatment: a retrospective cohort study of children, adolescents and young adults using the general practice research database. Drug Saf 32(11):1089–1096

Nicoli M, Bouchez S, Nieto I, Gasquet I, Kovess V, Lepine JP (2012) Prevalence and risk factors for suicide ideation, plans and attempts in the French general population: results from the ESEMeD study. Encéphale 38(4):296–303

Nordstrom P et al (1994) CSF 5-HIAA predicts suicide risk after attempted suicide. Suicide Life Threat Behav 24(1):1–9

Ozdemir E, Karaman MG, Yurteri N, Erdogan A (2010) A case of suicide attempt with long-acting methylphenidate (Concerta). Atten Defic Hyperact Disord 2(3):103–105

Polanczyk G, de Lima MS, Horta BL, Biederman J, Rohde LA (2007) The worldwide prevalence of ADHD: a systematic review and metaregression analysis. Am J Psychiatry 164(6):942–948

Putnins AL (2005) Correlates and predictors of self-reported suicide attempts among incarcerated youths. Int J Offender Ther Comp Criminol 49(2):143–157

Santosh PJ, Sattar S, Canagaratnam M (2011) Efficacy and tolerability of pharmacotherapies for attention-deficit hyperactivity disorder in adults. CNS Drugs 25(9):737–763

Sharav VH (2003) The impact of the food and drug administration modernization act on the recruitment of children for research. Ethical Hum Sci Serv 5(2):83–108

Swann AC, Steinberg JL, Lijffijt M, Moeller FG (2008) Impulsivity: differential relationship to depression and mania in bipolar disorder. J Affect Disord 106(3):241–248. Epub

Wilens TE, Adler LA, Adams J, Sgambati S, Rotrosen J, Sawtelle R, Utzinger L, Fusillo S (2008) Misuse and diversion of stimulants prescribed for ADHD: a systematic review of the literature. J Am Acad Child Adolesc Psychiatry 47(1):21–31. doi:10.1097/chi.0b013e31815a56f1, Review. PubMed PMID: 18174822

www.caddra.ca

ADHD and Alcohol/Substance Use Disorder

5

Objectives

1. Describe the prevalence and epidemiology of ADHD and substance/alcohol use disorder
2. Explain the link between ADHD and SUD
3. Describe some of the challenges in the diagnostic assessment of ADHD and SUD
4. List some of the psychiatric disorders that should be considered and included in the differential diagnosis when assessing individuals with substance use disorders
5. Recognize some of the barriers to seeking addiction treatment
6. Describe tools and approaches that health professionals can use to screen for and diagnose alcohol use disorder
7. Describe some of the management considerations that clinicians should recognize when using ADHD medications in individuals with ADHD and addictions
8. Describe some of the factors that help make the decision of how long to wait for SUD to be under control before initiating pharmacological treatment of adult ADHD
9. Understand the treatment recommendations for substance abusing patients with ADHD
10. Describe the epidemiology, morbidity, and common reasons for stimulant abuse and diversion

5.1 The Case of Sam Small

Sam Small is a 25-year-old single white male who is a second year student in the plumbing program at the Local Community College in Halifax, Nova Scotia, Canada. He also works part time as an apprentice plumber in a plumbing company. He lives close to his community college but his hometown is Ottawa, Canada. He has no family in Halifax.

© Springer International Publishing Switzerland 2017
J. Sadek, *Clinician's Guide to Adult ADHD Comorbidities*,
DOI 10.1007/978-3-319-39794-8_5

When asked for the reason for his visit, Sam reports "My ADHD medications are not working anymore so I stopped it. I cannot sleep and I need a prescription for marijuana. It is the only thing that helps me sleep." He also mentioned increased irritability and anger.

History of Present Illness Sam mentioned that the past 3 months had been very difficult. He had to work most weekends because of a pressure from his boss. His program has been very demanding and he was assaulted recently but refused to talk about it and he mentioned that he never went to the police. He said that his Adderrall (mixed amphetamine salts) stopped working so he stopped taking the medication 3 weeks ago. He has been prescribed 40 mg daily in the morning but he said that the medication was not working anymore. He has been taking it for the past 3 years and previously was prescribed MPH.

Mood Symptoms Screening He tells you, "*Over the past 10 days, my mood has been really irritable most of the time. It is getting more and more difficult to complete my course work on time, and I am not making any progress on my work.*" When asked why, he says, "*It's partly because my energy is so low… and partly because I just don't care. I have been missing lots of time in school in the mornings because I don't wake up, and when I wake up, I often feel sick*". When you ask about his symptoms he says, "*Well, mostly headaches, and often I feel nauseous. Sometimes I vomit. But I usually feel better later in the day.*" He denies having any current thoughts of suicide. He enjoys music and watching movies. He has many friends and he denied grandiose thoughts or behavior. His speech is not rapid and he does not talk much. He has middle insomnia but he compensates by sleeping during the day. He denied recent changes in his behavior.

Anxiety Screening Sam worries about his school, his finances, and his relationship with his boss. He is able to control his worries. He denied having panic episodes. Sam has no specific phobias and denies symptoms of OCD and PTSD.

Psychosis Screening Sam denies active hallucinations and his mental status examination shows no formal thought disorder and no delusions. No active psychotic symptoms and no history of psychosis.

Alcohol Screen As part of your assessment, you ask Sam to complete the CAGE questionnaire. Although he denies ever feeling that he needed to cut down on his drinking, or feeling guilty about his drinking, He does admit that some of his roommates have told him to cut back on his drinking. They also told him that they have felt annoyed by some of his behaviors when he is drinking. He also admits to frequently having a beer shortly after getting up in the morning as, "*This is the best way to take my sick feeling away.*" Sam is somewhat evasive in his answers and tries to avoid the topic. After detailed questioning, he admits that he first began drinking at age 15 while in high school and was a light frequent drinker at that time.

Currently, he has at least four drinks every day but from Thursday to Sunday He usually has 6–8 drinks a day. He said *"I don't really care what I drink, but I prefer beer and vodka. Over the past few months, though, I've mostly been drinking vodka. When I came to College, I didn't drink much. I guess I drank once every two weeks, and usually only one or two drinks at a time. But things change when in this College. It's what you do to unwind and meet people, and I'm no different. So, I've been drinking like I do now for almost a year."*

Sam tells you that he was caught once drinking while driving. He also admits that he had a visit to the emergency room once when his friends took him after he passed out during a party, but that everything was OK and he was released when he woke up. He admits that he did have a number of nondrinking friends when he first arrived at College, but he doesn't see them anymore. Sam maintains again that all of his friends drink now, and many of them use other drugs from time to time. He doesn't feel he has a problem.

Other Substance Use Screening   In exploring further Sam's substance use, he tells you, *"I suppose I use marijuana three to four times a week, usually one joint each time. I've tried ecstasy four or five times at parties."* He said that marijuana has been helping him to sleep so now he is using two joints each time he uses.

You asked about his stimulant use. He was very reluctant to answer but he said that since work and school became very demanding, he needed to "double up" on his stimulant medication so he ran out and the pharmacy refused to dispense the remainder of his prescription because he was 3 weeks early. He mentioned that his headaches increased and he feels his heart is going so fast when he was taking double the amount. He said he is frequently approached on campus with people offering him other stimulant medications but he has not being buying.

Medical History   Sam denies any current active medical problems. He had an appendectomy at age 15. He is healthy. His physical examination is unremarkable. He has no drug allergy.

Family History   When asked about his family history, he tells you that his father has high cholesterol. He has an aunt with diabetes and another paternal aunt who committed suicide a year ago. His father and his brother (his uncle) have alcohol addiction problems, but he says that his father has been sober for 4 years. His mother has been diagnosed with depression and was admitted to a psychiatric hospital 4 years ago when she was treated with ECT (electroconvulsive therapy). He has two brothers (one age 20 and one age 11). His 11-year-old brother has ADHD inattentive type and was started on MPH (methylphenidate) long acting.

Personal History   You ask about his childhood. *"My childhood was OK, but Mom and Dad fought a lot, mostly around Dad's drinking. My parents went through a hard time but were able to continue together.* He said his parents were not rich but his needs were met. He tells you that he talks with his mom on the phone or by Skype at least three times a week. His relationship with his father is more distant. He denied history of sexual abuse but he was physically abused and bullied in school. He started having a tear in his eye when he admits to bullying, but he is unwilling to talk about it any further. He says that he never failed a grade in school but the report cards mentioned "hyperactivity," "not waiting his turn to answer questions," "day dreaming," "not reaching his potential," and not finishing his work. He had few close friends and used to be very involved in different sports. He said he wishes to go back to sports and wishes he can join the college's football team. He used to work in a coffee shop part time for many years and he enjoyed that job. After finishing grade 12, he worked for 3 years full time but decided to go back to school part time and was accepted in Halifax, so he moved from Ontario to join the community college.

He was not aware of any community resources and never been to any local center that deals with addictions. Sam has no spiritual or religious beliefs or affiliation. He has no criminal record.

Sam recently broke up with his last girlfriend because she was asking him to stop drinking and using weed. Sam became very sad when he talked about the break up with his girlfriend. He said "she really cared, she was very nice and kind...I still love her. She is the best and I wish I could get her back".

At this point, he appears somewhat reflective, and tells you, "*I don't know why things have changed so much in my life.*" You take advantage of the comment and try to do a brief intervention. You ask him empathetically if he can make a possible link between his drinking and his falling grades, loss of his girlfriend, and changes in his lifestyle. He is able to see the link. You ask him about the advantages of quitting versus using but he quickly cuts you off by saying, "My drinking is not the problem. I'm like most of the college students. "It's not a problem for me." You are about to get annoyed but you recognize that the resistance is active and you try to roll with the resistance by summarizing his current use and problems and comparing them to his goals of finishing college, having a good career, and getting his girlfriend back. You give him clear advice and say "your drinking is more than what is medically safe". "I strongly recommend that you quit and I am willing to help".

You suggest to him that he may benefit from admission to the Detox center. He felt that you are sincere in trying to help him. He said "give me the number, I will give them a call." He calls the Detox from your office and luckily they have a bed. He leaves your office and goes right to the Detox center.

Sam was discharged one week later and came for a follow up visit. He was discharged on trazodone 50 mg at bedtime for sleep and a small dose of benzodiazepine that is being tapered. He felt that the admission was very helpful. He is motivated to stay sober and hopes to start doing well in school. You scheduled a weekly appointment and he agreed to urine drug screening each visit.

5.1.1   Visit 3

In his third visit, he mentioned that he is attending school regularly. He is back to his normal work routine but really struggling with his ADHD symptoms that he had all his life. His ADHD diagnosis has been confirmed from the reports of his family doctor that he sent from Ontario. He was diagnosed with ADHD combined type at age 7 and he had a psychoeducational assessment in school. He was tried on different medications until high school when he stopped them. His hyperactivity symptoms improved but symptoms of inattention persisted. He struggled to obtain grade 12 but when he started college, his family doctor restarted him on Adderrall 10 mg in the morning and the dose increased to 40 mg AM by the end of the first year that he successfully completed. Patient reported the following difficulties that he consider very severe and interfere with his function:

Shifting from one uncompleted task to another, difficulty with tasks that require memory, poor use of time and procrastinating, losing his tools at work and frequently buying new tools from his pocket, not listening to the instructions from his boss, staring off into space and that led him to making serious errors, difficulty sustaining attention in school particularly when instructors are giving details about specific projects. He said he is easily distracted by any sound or movement. He said that his work space is always messy and his car is extremely messy that people cannot get a ride with him because of all the clutter on the seats. He gave consent to talk to his parents who both confirmed that he has a long history of ADHD that truly impairs his functioning. Sam said that the past year has been a dark period in his life and he does not wish to return to alcohol or drugs anymore. He regrets misusing his stimulants and felt that doubling the dose had been very scary, and at one point he felt his heart was going so fast that he will die. He promised to follow medical advice and continue treatment.

Review of the Literature Questions
Epidemiology, Etiology, and Morbidity Questions

Describe the prevalence and epidemiology of ADHD and Substance/Alcohol Use Disorder?

Comorbidity of substance use disorder and ADHD is high. Substance use disorders are common in adolescents and adults with ADHD, and some studies suggested that 33 % of adult ADHD patients were having a history of an alcohol use disorder and 20 % were having a drug use disorder [1], [2]. Literature also suggests that one-quarter of adults with SUDs, and one-half of adolescents with SUDs, have ADHD. Adults with SUDs also show a higher risk for ADHD, as well as earlier onset, and more severe SUDs, associated with ADHD [2].

ADHD significantly increased the risk for alcohol abuse, cannabis abuse, and other illicit substances, in both males and females, compared to individuals without ADHD [3].

The misuse of marijuana, alcohol, or the combination of the two are the most common substances of abuse in adolescents with ADHD but one important antecedent to developing SUD in children and adolescents with ADHD is cigarette smoking. Cocaine and stimulant abuse is not overrepresented in ADHD; but marijuana continues to be the most commonly abused agent [4].

Explain the Link Between ADHD and SUD?

The self-medication hypothesis is plausible in ADHD. Moreover, the accompanying poor self-judgment and impulsivity associated with ADHD may be conducive to the development of SUD.

The second hypothesis relies on neurobiological link. Functional imaging studies have demonstrated that there may be deficits in anterior cingulate activation and the frontosubcortical systems, in both individuals with ADHD and SUD.

Genetic and family research support the link between ADHD and SUD. It appears that exposure to nicotine, alcohol or substances during pregnancy increases the risk of development of ADHD in the offspring. Literature also has shown that siblings, parents, and offspring of individuals with SUD share the etiologies of ADHD and SUD as well as several genes.

Comorbid disorders may also support the link between ADHD and SUD. Co-occurring conduct or bipolar disorders increase risk of SUD among ADHD patients. Some controversy exists about the relationship between ADHD treatment and substance use [5].

Describe some of the challenges in the diagnostic assessment of ADHD and SUD?

Substance effects during acute intoxication or withdrawal may produce overlapping symptoms with ADHD such as impulsivity, agitation, mood instability, intolerance to frustrations, restlessness, concentration, and memory difficulties.

Craving and loss of control which are common part of the addictive process may also overlap with ADHD with symptoms of impulsivity, poor decision making, planning difficulties, mood instability, and continued substance use in spite of adverse consequences.

Deficits in executive function may be preexisting in both patients of ADHD and SUD with symptoms of impulsivity, risk-taking behavior, inattention, and inability to inhibit responses.

Common psychiatric comorbidities to addictions such as mood and anxiety disorders, borderline personality disorder, and antisocial personality disorder may show several overlapping symptoms of ADHD such as impulsivity, risk-taking behavior, and intolerance to frustration [6, 7].

What psychiatric disorders should be considered and included in the differential diagnosis when assessing individuals with substance use disorders?

Mood disorders (both unipolar depression and bipolar disorder), anxiety disorders, ADHD, personality disorders (borderline and antisocial), effect of substance (withdrawal, intoxication), sleep disorders such as obstructive sleep apnea, endocrine and metabolic disorders such as thyroid disorders, and neurological disorders (traumatic brain injury) [5].

What are some of the barriers to seeking Addiction treatment?

Major barriers to addiction treatment include:

- Stigma: perhaps one of the largest obstacle. In society, there is significant shame and stigma around addiction issues, where it remains viewed by many as a moral failing or lack of self-control. As a result, people are very hesitant to seek appropriate treatment, or do so in secrecy which is often unhelpful as it exacerbates the shame and increases the risk of relapse.
- Lack of appropriate resources – particularly in rural areas, there may be very limited treatment options. Larger areas have more resources, but may not be easily accessible.

- Unrecognized or untreated mental illness: psychosis, anxiety, depression, or other mental health issues may prevent patients from seeking treatment, as they attempt to "self-medicate" their psychological symptoms with mood altering substances. Similarly, if they do seek treatment for addiction issues and these comorbid conditions are not addressed, this dramatically worsens their prognosis and increases the risk of relapse.
- Primary support network that also use or abuse substances: many people find that those close to them in fact enable their ongoing substance use, and find it difficult to create a new support network of those who are supportive of positive change in their lives.
- Cost of treatment for patients who have limited income or unable to access public resources.
- Fear of consequences particularly if there are concerns that they may lose custody of their children, or if addiction treatment may be used against them in some manner.
- Ethnicity, culture, and gender specific issues: In some areas in the USA and Canada, the majority of those who seek treatment are Caucasian. Some cultural issues might also contribute to help seeking behavior. Gender specific issues particularly for women have been widely discussed in the literature.
- Lack of insight: many patients with addictions do not acknowledge that there is a problem so they do not seek help. Motivation enhancement techniques can be very helpful in these situations. Motivational interview is a method for enhancing motivation by exploring and resolving ambivalence. The principles of motivational interviewing include: asking open-ended questions, providing patient affirmation, practicing reflective listening, and summarizing [7, 9]

What models of care are used to treat concurrent disorders in patients with substance abuse? What are the strengths and weaknesses of these models?

Three primary models of service delivery exist for concurrent disorders:

1. Sequential treatment

   In sequential treatment, the individual seeks treatment for one disorder. Then – having successfully addressed that disorder – the patient moves on to treatment for the second disorder. The more serious or severe condition, viewed as the primary disorder, is generally tackled first. This approach may delay much-needed interventions.

   Most often, a person's two conditions are interrelated, so it can be very difficult to address the issues in isolation from one another. For example, addressing a drinking problem in someone who is profoundly depressed presents a serious clinical challenge. Often, sequential treatment results in neither condition receiving adequate or timely treatment. In this type of sequential approach, patients often end up going from one service to the other repeatedly, a frustrating experience that can cause them to give up on treatment entirely.

2. Parallel treatment

   In this model, individuals are cared for with a coordinated clinical care approach, one which addresses both mental health issues and addictions concerns together, drawing on the strengths and expertise of both types of clinical approaches. Mental health issues are tackled by those on the mental health team. At the same time, substance use issues are addressed by addictions staff. This type of treatment helps improve the individual's likelihood of successful recovery. The challenge to success in this model, however, is effective communication between caregivers. With multiple professionals involved, an accountability system is needed to ensure that clinicians communicate regularly with one another and not give conflicting advice or messages to patients based on differing treatment practices and philosophies.

3. Integrated treatment

In this model, patients receive treatment for all their addiction and mental health conditions under the care of a single multidisciplinary team. The theory behind this treatment model is that one cohesive team simultaneously addressing all aspects of mental health and addictions may improve outcomes [10].

List some useful screening tools for Alcohol Disorder?

Several screening tools are available in the literature.

One of the most common screening tools is the CAGE:

C – Have you ever tried to cut down your drinking?
A – Have people annoyed you by criticizing your drinking?
G – Have you ever felt bad or guilty about your drinking?
E – Have you ever had a drink first thing in the morning to steady your nerves or to help a hangover? ("eye-opener")

Other possible instruments include:

AUDIT: Alcohol Use Disorder Identification Test
ASSIST: Alcohol, Smoking, and Substance Involvement Screening Test
S-MAST: Short Michigan Alcohol Screening Test
RAPS: Rapid Alcohol Problems Screening
FAST: Fast Alcohol Screening Tool for Emergency Room.

Describe some on the management considerations that clinicians should recognize when using ADHD medications in individuals with ADHD and addictions?

ADHD medications appear to have little to no efficacy in the treatment of comorbid addictive disorders but do not appear to exacerbate addictive disorders. Majority of the controlled clinical trials did not find enough evidence of exacerbation but it should be noted that a few cases of abuse and misuse have been reported in uncontrolled clinical studies.

ADHD medications appear less effective in ADHD patients with addictive disorders compared to patients without these comorbid disorders. It appears that although the various medications (both stimulants and nonstimulants) assessed in several studies can improve ADHD in the short term, they are less effective in ADHD patients with addictive disorders than in patients without these comorbid disorders.

Researchers challenge the available evidence and consider it ambiguous in terms of whether differences in adherence affect clinical outcomes in patients treated for adult ADHD.

ADHD medications seem to exert a strong placebo effect on ADHD symptoms in patients with addictive disorders. Some studies report placebo response rates as high as 45–55 %. The high placebo response may be related to a nonspecific effect of addiction treatment on impulsivity and aggressiveness. Such an effect probably lessens the severity of some clinical manifestations of ADHD. Another possible explanation may be related to the high expectations of patients with addictions or their treating clinicians that medical treatment will improve ADHD symptoms.

Possibly the concomitant psychosocial treatment (mainly cognitive behavioral therapy) to many of the controlled studies may have contributed to the reported efficacy of the ADHD medications.

Some researchers suggest that ADHD and SUD-related craving share neurobiological similarities, and that treatment of ADHD may reduce craving for substances and subsequently reduce the risk for relapse to substance use. An aggregate of the literature seems to suggest that early stimulant treatment reduces, or delays, the onset of SUDs and perhaps cigarette smoking into adolescence; however, the protective effect is lost in adulthood. These issues remain unclear and further research is needed in these areas.

Describe some of the factors that help make the decision of how long to wait for SUD to be under control before initiating pharmacological treatment of adult ADHD.

The relationship between ADHD and SUD is bidirectional. The decision to treat or not treat ADHD in the context of active substance abuse depends on numerous factors. Among these are:

1. The type and severity of substance involved
2. The patient's opinion about the importance of ADHD in his/her particular case
3. The degree of diagnostic uncertainty for ADHD
4. The risk of exacerbating SUD and other mental disorders by treating ADHD
5. The experience of the treatment team in the management of SUD and ADHD comorbidity
6. The ability to closely monitor the patient's adherence and response to treatment

It is recommended to individualize the treatment decision due to the multiple challenges of ADHD and SUD comorbidity. The decision should be done on a case-by-case basis in which the arguments for and against immediate pharmacological treatment of ADHD are carefully weighed. The results of such an assessment will indicate when to initiate ADHD treatment and the most appropriate choice of medication.

What are the treatment recommendations for substance abusing patients with ADHD?

The strategy for caring for patients with SUD and ADHD should include consideration of both disorders. A complete assessment of the substance use and

ADHD needs be conducted prior to treatment. Once the substance use is better controlled or in a harm reduction model, the uses of psychotherapeutic intervention such as motivational interviewing and CBT appear to be useful as a first step for addressing both the ADHD and SUD. They would incorporate structured and goal-directed sessions as well as active therapist involvement. Additionally, pharmacological agents can be used in conjunction with psychotherapy in order to alleviate ADHD symptoms and further substance use. Psycho-education is also useful. Furthermore, young adults with SUD benefit from both family and individual intervention.

Several review studies have suggested that the use of nonstimulant agents (atomoxetine), antidepressants (bupropion), and extended-release or longer acting stimulants with lower abuse liability and diversion potential is preferable when treating patients with comorbid ADHD and SUD.

For patients with ADHD and an ongoing SUD or a recent history of SUD, nonstimulant treatment with atomoxetine may be preferred.

There have been some differences in the literature regarding response to atomoxetine depending upon the time the treatment was initiated (e.g., whether the study subjects were actively engaging in substance abuse or dependence versus being engaged in brief abstinence). Further research is also needed in these areas [5].

Stimulant Medications Abuse, Misuse, and Diversion

Describe some of the concepts related to stimulant medications abuse and misuse?

Stimulant medications, like illicit psychostimulants, have the potential to induce abuse and dependence. Along with opioids and central nervous system depressants, stimulants are one of the most commonly abused pharmaceutical drug classes. Some evidence for the abuse liability of pharmaceutical stimulants can be found in both animal and human research. Stimulant-induced elevations in brain dopamine appear to be integral to both efficacy in ADHD and potential for abuse [11].

These stimulant medications, particularly when injected or in immediate-release form, could produce subjective and reinforcing effects similar to the illicit psychostimulants.

Some researchers argued that much of the concern about these medications is based on reports of "misuse," rather than "abuse." Misuse can range from noncompliance to compulsive abuse [12, 13].

What is the rate of stimulants misuse or abuse in high school students versus university and college ?

Among US and Canadian school students, the reported prevalence of past year pharmaceutical stimulant misuse is 5–9 %, and past year methylphenidate use 2–5 %. Studies of stimulant misuse among university/college students have yielded life-time prevalence estimates of 7–17 %, and 5–35 % for past year. One recent study of misuse has found life-time prevalence rates of 5–43 % and past year prevalence rates of 5–6 % and misuse peak prevalence from 16 to 24 years of age, with a decline over subsequent years. Stimulant medications misuse or abuse is more prevalent on university/college campuses than among young adults in the general population. In one study, students aged 18–22 years were found to be more than twice as likely to report misuse of MPH in the past year (6.4 % versus 3.0 %). Mixed amphet-amine salts were more likely to have been misused among college students than nonstudent peers (7.9 % versus 5.4 %), [11–13].

What are the correlates of Diversion and misuse?

1. Higher rates of hyperactivity–impulsivity
2. Conduct disorder
3. Other illicit drug use
4. Male
5. Caucasian
6. A college or university attendee [11]

Describe some of the research findings on stimulant medications diversion?

There are few studies that have reported specifically on diversion. Research [4] found reports of diversion in six of the studies they reviewed, with life-time rates of diversion ranging from 11 to 29 %. Personal experience of diversion appears far less prevalent than knowledge of diversion among others. Sharp & Rosen found that, while only 8 % of students had sold or given away medication themselves, 63 % knew someone else who had done so, and 67 % knew someone who had taken stimulant medication recreationally. Other studies have measured the prevalence of students with prescriptions being asked to sell, trade, or give away their medication, with 23–84 % of students having been approached [4, 14].

What are the reasons of abuse or misuse of stimulant medications?

1. To improve attention, concentration and alertness, study habits, and academic performance
2. Pleasure seeking and to get high
3. Craving
4. Habits or impulsivity [14, 15].

What are the clinical implications of stimulants abuse or diversion?

Those diverting ADHD medication are not receiving the full benefits of pharmacotherapy and those receiving diverted medication are placing themselves at unnecessary risk of adverse health effects or toxicity [14].

References

1. Kessler RC, Nelson CB, McGonagle KA, Edlund MJ, Frank RG, Leaf PJ (1996) The epidemiology of co-occurring addictive and mental disorders: implications for prevention and service utilization. Am J Orthopsychiatry 66(1):17–31.
2. Wilens TE, Adler LA, Adams J, Sgambati S, Rotrosen J, Sawtelle R, Utzinger L, Fusillo S (2008) Misuse and diversion of stimulants prescribed for ADHD: a systematic review of the literature. J Am Acad Child Adolesc Psychiatry 47(1):21–31. doi: 10.1097/chi.0b013e31815a56f1.
3. Ottosen C, Petersen L, Larsen JT, Dalsgaard S (2016) Gender differences in associations between attention-deficit/hyperactivity disorder and substance use disorder. J Am Acad Child Adolesc Psychiatry 55(3):227–234.e4

4. Wilens TE et al (2011) Does ADHD predict substance-use disorders? A 10-year follow-up study of young adults with ADHD. J Am Acad Child Adolesc Psychiatry 50(6):543–553
5. Zulauf CA, Sprich SE, Safren SA, Wilens TE (2014) The complicated relationship between attention deficit/hyperactivity disorder and substance use disorders. Curr Psychiatry Rep 16(3):436
6. Fatseas M, Debrabant R, Auriacombe M (2012) The diagnostic accuracy of attention-deficit/ hyperactivity disorder in adults with substance use disorders. Curr Opin Psychiatry 25(3): 219–225
7. Fatseas M, Debrabant R, Auriacombe M (2012) The diagnostic accuracy of attention-deficit/ hyperactivity disorder in adults with substance use disorders. Curr Opin Psychiatry 25(3):219–225. doi:10.1097/YCO.0b013e3283523d7c. Review
8. Probst C, Manthey J, Martinez A, Rehm J (2015) Alcohol use disorder severity and reported reasons not to seek treatment: a cross-sectional study in European primary care practices. Subst Abuse Treat Prev Policy 10:32
9. Saunders SM, Zygowicz KM, D'Angelo BR (2006) Person-related and treatment-related barriers to alcohol treatment. J Subst Abuse Treat 30(3):261–270
10. Torrens M, Rossi PC, Martinez-Riera R, Martinez-Sanvisens D, Bulbena A (2012) Psychiatric co-morbidity and substance use disorders: treatment in parallel systems or in one integrated system? Subst Use Misuse 47(8–9):1005–1014
11. Clemow DB, Walker DJ (2014) The potential for misuse and abuse of medications in ADHD: a review. Postgrad Med 126(5):64–81. doi:10.3810/pgm.2014.09.2801. Review
12. Kollins SH (2008) A qualitative review of issues arising in the use of psycho-stimulant medications in patients with ADHD and co-morbid substance use disorders. Curr Med Res Opin 24(5):1345–1357
13. Kollins SH (2008) A qualitative review of issues arising in the use of psycho-stimulant medications in patients with ADHD and co-morbid substance use disorders. Curr Med Res Opin 24(5):1345–1357. doi:10.1185/030079908X280707. Epub 2008 Apr 1. Review
14. Rabiner DL (2013) Stimulant prescription cautions: addressing misuse, diversion and malingering. Curr Psychiatry Rep 15(7):375. doi:10.1007/s11920-013-0375-2. Review
15. Newton TF (2009) Theories of addiction: methamphetamine users' explanations for continuing drug use and relapse. Am J Addict 18:294–300

Bibliography

Clay SW, Allen J, Parran T (2008) A review of addiction. Postgrad Med 120(2):E01–E07
Emmerik-van Oortmerssen K, van de Glind G et al (2014) Psychiatric comorbidity in treatment-seeking substance use disorder patients with and without attention deficit hyperactivity disorder: results of the IASP study. Addiction 109(2):262–272
Harstad E, Levy S, Committee on Substance Abuse (2014) Attention-deficit/hyperactivity disorder and substance abuse. Pediatrics 134(1):e293–e301. doi:10.1542/peds.2014-0992. Review
Jones LA (2011) Systematic review of alcohol screening tools for use in the emergency department. Emerg Med J 28(3):182–191
Kaye S, Darke S (2012) The diversion and misuse of pharmaceutical stimulants: what do we know and why should we care? Addiction 107(3):467–477. doi:10.1111/j.1360-0443.2011.03720.x. Review
Klassen LJ, Bilkey TS, Katzman MA, Chokka P (2012) Comorbid attention deficit/hyperactivity disorder and substance use disorder: treatment considerations. Curr Drug Abuse Rev 5(3):190–198. Review
Levin FR (2007) Diagnosing attention-deficit/hyperactivity disorder in patients with substance use disorders. J Clin Psychiatry 68(Suppl 11):9–14. Review
Murthy P, Chand P (2012) Treatment of dual diagnosis disorders. Curr Opin Psychiatry 25(3):194–200. doi:10.1097/YCO.0b013e328351a3e0. Review

Retz W, Retz-Junginger P (2014) Prediction of methylphenidate treatment outcome in adults with attention-deficit/hyperactivity disorder (ADHD). Eur Arch Psychiatry Clin Neurosci 264(Suppl 1):S35–S43. doi:10.1007/s00406-014-0542-4. Epub 2014 Sep 18. Review

Spencer TJ (2009) Issues in the management of patients with complex attention-deficit hyperactivity disorder symptoms. CNS Drugs 23(Suppl1):9–20. doi:10.2165/00023210-200923000-00003. Review

Spencer TJ (2009) Issues in the management of patients with complex attention-deficit hyperactivity disorder symptoms. CNS Drugs 23(Suppl1):9–20

Upadhyaya HP (2007) Managing attention-deficit/hyperactivity disorder in the presence of substance use disorder. J Clin Psychiatry 68(Suppl 11):23–30. Review

Wilens TE (2007) The nature of the relationship between attention-deficit/hyperactivity disorder and substance use. J Clin Psychiatry 68(Suppl 11):4–8. Review

Wilens TE, Fusillo S (2007) When ADHD and substance use disorders intersect: relationship and treatment implications. Curr Psychiatry Rep 9(5):408–414. Review

Wilens TE, Upadhyaya HP (2007) Impact of substance use disorder on ADHD and its treatment. J Clin Psychiatry 68(8):e20. Review

Wolf LE, Simkowitz P, Carlson H (2009) College students with attention-deficit/hyperactivity disorder. Curr Psychiatry Rep 11(5):415–421. Review

ADHD and Bipolar Disorder

6

Objectives

1. Describe the prevalence, epidemiology, and morbidity of ADHD and bipolar disorder
2. Recognize some of the overlapping and differentiating features between ADHD and Bipolar Disorder
3. Understand the current literature recommendations for treating Bipolar disorder comorbid with ADHD

6.1   The Case of Bonnie Boston

Bonnie Boston is a 25-year-old female who lives with her 32-year-old husband. She works in a restaurant. She has no children. She has a diagnosis of ADHD and Bipolar disorder.

Reason for the Visit Bonnie decided to go back to school to become a pharmacy technician. She has been off her ADHD medications since age 18 when she finished high school. Now she is requesting to start ADHD treatment.

6.2   History of Present Illness and Review of Systems

Bonnie endorses short-term memory problems and requires daily reminders. Without her Blackberry she would never remember appointments. Her room and car are described as messy. She has chronic problems with attention to detail saying, "every time I fill out a form, it gets sent back because it is incomplete." She struggles to sustain attention for more than 10 min while doing boring tasks. She tends to avoid tasks that require sustained mental effort. She misplaces her keys, glasses and ID badge all the time. To combat this she has chosen a spot on the hall table where she keeps her keys so she can find them. She is often easily distracted. As a child,

© Springer International Publishing Switzerland 2017
J. Sadek, *Clinician's Guide to Adult ADHD Comorbidities*,
DOI 10.1007/978-3-319-39794-8_6

her teachers often commented that she was a daydreamer. Comments on old report cards stated: "not finishing her homework…not paying attention…day dreaming… not reaching her potential". She is considered a hyperactive individual and her impulsive behaviours involve substance use, sex and shopping sprees.

Bonnie described her mood as great. She denied suicidal thoughts and she never attempted. She takes Melatonin 5 mg for sleep. No problems with appetite. She described her concentration as poor and her attention span is short. Her energy is very good. She complains of poor motivation, procrastinating, and she is overwhelmed by expectations. She enjoys listening to music and dancing. She never had psychotic symptoms

In terms of anxiety, Bonnie said, "I worry about everything. I worry about people criticizing me" She does not experience panic attacks. She can control her worries.

Bonnie was asked about her substance and alcohol use. She said she binge drinks approximately once every 2 or 3 weeks. She has used marijuana since age 17 but stopped it at age 19. She said she tried cocaine twice in high school.

6.3   Past Psychiatric History

Bonnie has had two admissions to hospital over the past 5 years with diagnoses of substance abuse, bipolar disorder and ADHD. Her first admission was for bipolar depression and her second admission she had a manic episode.

She has been prescribed many psychiatric medications. She has been on a combination of medications including fluoxetine 20 mg and lamotregne 100 mg HS, lithium 900 mg HS and venlfaxine 225 mg daily, quetiapine 400 mg HS and bupropion 300 mg daily. She had significant weight gain with lamotrigine so she stopped it. Because of her back pain, she took lots of Ibuprofen that contributed to toxic Lithium level and poor kidney function. Lithium was stopped and her kidney function returned to normal. Quetiapine was associated with 18 Lbs weight gain so she stopped it. Currently she is maintained on Epival (divalproex sodium 1250 mg at bedtime). At age 10 she was prescribed long acting mixed amphetamine salt but when her parents separated, her father was no longer able to afford the medication therefore it was stopped.

6.4   Medical History

Bonnie has chronic back pain, peptic ulcer and is being investigated for polycystic ovary syndrome. She has allergies to penicillin and ASA. She had two abortions.

6.5   Family Medical and Psychiatric History

Bonnie has one older sister. Paternal grandparents abused alcohol. Her paternal grandmother, sister, and uncle have been diagnosed with depression. Her father also suffers from anxiety. Her mother has bipolar disorder and they do not talk since she left the family when Bonnie was 14 years old.

6.6   Personal History

Bennie's mother smoked cigarettes while pregnant with her, but consumed no drugs or alcohol. Bonnie was born by caesarean section. Developmental milestones were achieved in due time. She was described as an emotional child who was accident-prone. She had chronic sleep problems since she was a child.

During elementary school she received average marks and was often disruptive. In spite of this she seemed to get along reasonably well with other children and teachers. School performance dropped in high school and she failed grade 11 and dropped out for 1 year but went back finished grade 12.

She has three close friends that she kept since she was a child. She enjoys social-izing with them. She started working at Wal-Mart at age 18 but hated her job. She enjoys working in her current restaurant.

Bonnie is very artistic and has won a number of awards for her works of art and dance performances.

She has been with her husband for the past 5 years.

6.7   Collateral Information from her Boyfriend

He confirmed that Bonnie has feelings of inner restlessness, agitation and has ten-dency to take risks. She gets bored easily and has trouble sitting still and she is constantly fidgeting. She talks excessively likes doing too many things at once.

She frequently interrupt others and blurt out thoughts that are rude or inappropri-ate without thinking. She has trouble starting and finishing projects and usually she is late for work. She frequently forgets appointments, commitments, and deadlines and underestimating the time it will take you to complete tasks. He said her last manic episode was 3 years ago and she did not have any manic or depressive epi-sodes since then.

Impression and Plan Bipolar I disorder, ADHD, SUD in full sustained remission.

Since urine toxicology screen was negative and she is euthymic and stable on her Divalproex sodium and her blood level was at therapeutic level, patient was started on Methylphenidate 30 mg long acting po AM and was referred to a psychologist for psychosocial management of her ADHD and Bipolar illness.

6.7.1   Visit 2

Patient was brought by her husband 3 weeks later for urgent visit. She decided to stop her Divalproex sodium and was taking 60 mg daily of Methylphenidate Long acting.

Her husband found her up all night and started posting very rude and bizarre comments on Facebook. She said she can heal some types of cancer and she is able to bring her dead grandmother back to life with a soup. She went to the restaurant where she works and talked to the owner offering him to buy the restaurant for two million Dollars because she has an amazing project that will generate Billions of Dollars each year. The owner felt that Bonnie is acting in a very bizarre way so he called her husband immediately and her husband brought her to you.

You admitted Bonnie to the psychiatric acute care unit with diagnosis of Bipolar I mania with psychotic features. You stopped her MPH and started her on Olanzapine 10 mg AM and HS and restarted her on Divalproex sodium.

Literature Review Questions
Describe the prevalence, epidemiology and morbidity of ADHD and Bipolar Disorder?

The rates of comorbidity of ADHD and Bipolar disorder are high. The prevalence of bipolar disorder (BD) in children and adults with ADHD is elevated relative to non-ADHD peers. Some studies suggest that 5–20 % of adults with ADHD may also have BD [1, 2].

Other studies reported that 10–21 % of adults with BD may have comorbid ADHD [2, 3]. Because of similarities between symptom profiles, particularly if the developmental courses of the different disorders are not taken into account, pure ADHD or pure BD may be mistaken for comorbid ADHD-BD (and vice versa)

Comorbid ADHD and Bipolar Disorder patients experience:

- More severe mood episodes and more frequent affective episodes
- Earlier age of onset of Bipolar symptoms
- Shorter duration of wellness
- More suicide attempts
- More comorbid disorders particularly substance use disorder, Anxiety disorders and Antisocial Personality Disorder.
- More legal problems
- Reduced social functioning, educational achievements, employment rates and quality of life [2, 4, 5].

What are some of the overlapping features between ADHD and Bipolar Disorder?

ADHD symptom	Bipolar disorder symptom
Easily distracted by extraneous stimuli	Distractibility (attention too easily drawn to unimportant or irrelevant external stimuli)
Often 'on the go,' "acting as if 'driven by a motor'"	"Increase in goal-directed activity"
Often 'on the go,' "acting as if 'driven by a motor'"	Psychomotor agitation (i.e., purposeless non-goal directed activity).
Often talks excessively	More talkative than usual or pressure to keep talking
Often blurts out an answer before a question has been completed	More talkative than usual or pressure to keep talking
Often interrupts or intrudes on others	More talkative than usual or pressure to keep talking

(Asherson et al. [2]; Brus et al. [6])

Describe some of the differentiating features between ADHD and Bipolar Disorder?

ADHD symptom	Bipolar Disorder (BD) symptom
Continuous course	Episodic course, discrete period of illness
Several symptoms must be present before age 12	Rare in preadolescents
Severity does not often increase over time and possibly attenuate	Severity usually increase over time and cause more functional impairment over life cycle
Grandiosity is not apart of the ADHD symptom criteria	Grandiose thoughts or behaviour
No psychotic features	Psychotic features (such as delusions or hallucinations)
Poor sleep or delayed sleep phase usually not part of the diagnostic criteria	Decrease need of sleep is part of the manic episode
Elevated or expansive mood is not part of the diagnostic criteria	Elevated or expansive mood are part of the diagnostic criteria
Racing thoughts or flight of ideas is not part of the diagnostic criteria	Racing thoughts or flight of ideas are part of the diagnostic criteria
Not part of ADHD diagnosis	Increase in goal directed activity as spending money or sexual behavior
Restlessness	Increase in psychomotor activity or agitation

What are the management recommendations for treating Bipolar disorder comorbid with ADHD?

There is paucity of data describing treatment of Bipolar disorder (BD) comorbid with ADHD

As a general rule, Bipolar disorder should be treated first. Manic episodes are successfully treated with mood stabilizers, atypical antipsychotics or combinations. Psychotic features require aggressive antipsychotic treatment and Suicide should be assessed and managed as a priority

Stimulant medications should not be used in actively psychotic patents and if used in euythymic stable patient, they should be carefully monitored and evaluated.

Psychosocial treatment for DAHD should be emphasized in patients with comorbid BD and ADHD.

One author suggested that in the majority of patients, a hierarchical approach is desirable, with mood stabilization preceding the treatment of ADHD symptoms. Stimulants and atomoxetine in ADHD-BD comorbidity in adulthood and can be considered as possible options to be carefully evaluated once the patient has been stabilized and euthymic.

In an open-label study, adults with ADHD/BD who were taking BD medication (i.e., antipsychotics or mood stabilizers) were given bupropion to control ADHD symptoms. Compared to baseline, bupropion treatment significantly reduced ADHD symptoms, with no evidence of mania activation [7]. Bupropion has less manic switch rate than several antidepressants but continue to have the risk of mood destabilization.

Second generation antipsychotics may reduce the efficacy of dopamine-enhancing agents such as stimulants.

Response to mood stabilizers may be blunted in patients with ADHD.

Antidepressants Atomoxetine may also carry a small risk of switching Bipolar euthymic patients to mania. Atomoxetine should not be coadministered with SSRIs, which inhibit the cytochrome P450 2D6 isoenzyme because of the potential for pharmacokinetic interactions.

Few studies described use of psychostimulants in combination with mood-stabilizing drugs. Patients taking stable doses of mood stabilizers respond well to methylphenidate and amphetamine.

Drug-drug interactions are described between antiepileptic medications and MPH. Antiepileptic medications that act as mood stabilizers lower the level of methyphenidate and MPH may lower the effectiveness of these drugs.

References

1. Wingo AP, Ghaemi SN (2007) A systematic review of rates and diagnostic validity of comorbid adult attention-deficit/hyperactivity disorder and bipolar disorder. J Clin Psychiatry 68: 1776–1784
2. Asherson P, Young AH, Eich-Höchli D, Moran P, Porsdal V, Deberdt W (2014) Differential diagnosis, comorbidity, and treatment of attention-deficit/hyperactivity disorder in relation to bipolar disorder or borderline personality disorder in adults. Curr Med Res Opin 30(8):1657–1672
3. Tamam L, Karakus G, Ozpoyraz N (2008) Comorbidity of adult attention-deficit hyperactivity disorder and bipolar disorder: prevalence and clinical correlates. Eur Arch Psychiatry Clin Neurosci 258:385–393
4. Klassen LJ, Katzman MA, Chokka P (2010) Adult ADHD and its comorbidities, with a focus on bipolar disorder. J Affect Disord. 124(1–2):1–8.
5. Bond DJ, Hadjipavlou G, Lam RW, McIntyre RS, Beaulieu S, Schaffer A, Weiss M; Canadian Network for Mood and Anxiety Treatments (CANMAT) Task Force (2012) The Canadian Network for Mood and Anxiety Treatments (CANMAT) task force recommendations for the management of patients with mood disorders and comorbid attention-deficit/hyperactivity disorder. Ann Clin Psychiatry. 24(1):23–37. Review.
6. Brus MJ, Solanto MV, Goldberg JF (2014) Adult ADHD vs. bipolar disorder in the DSM-5 era: a challenging differentiation for clinicians. J Psychiatr Pract 20(6):428–437
7. Wilens TE, Prince JB, Spencer T, Van Patten SL, Doyle R, Girard K, Hammerness P, Goldman S, Brown S, Biederman J (2003) An open trial of bupropion for the treatment of adults with attention-deficit/hyperactivity disorder and bipolar disorder. Biol Psychiatry. 54(1):9–16

Bibliography

Perugi G, Vannucchi G (2015) The use of stimulants and atomoxetine in adults with comorbid ADHD and bipolar disorder. Expert Opin Pharmacother 16(14):2193–2204. doi:10.1517/1465 6566.2015.1079620. Review
Scheffer RE (2007) Concurrent ADHD and bipolar disorder. Curr Psychiatry Rep 9:415–419
Pacchiarotti I, Bond DJ, Baldessarini RJ et al (2013) The International Society for Bipolar Disorders (ISBD) task force report on antidepressant use in bipolar disorders. Am J Psychiatry 170(11):1249–1262
Corp SA, Gitlin MJ, Altshuler LL (2014) A review of the use of stimulants and stimulant alternatives in treating bipolar depression and major depressive disorder. J Clin Psychiatry 75(9):1010–1018

ADHD and Anxiety Disorders

7

Objectives
1. Describe the prevalence rates and some epidemiological data of ADHD and anxiety
2. List the overlapping and differentiating symptoms between ADHD and anxiety disorders
3. Describe some of the difficulties in conducting meta-analysis on the effect of stimulant medications on comorbid anxiety in ADHD patients in the current literature
4. List some of the instruments that would assist clinicians in identifying different anxiety disorders
5. Describe some of the treatment considerations when managing comorbid ADHD and anxiety disorders

7.1 The Case of Andrew Ashton

Identification A 39-year-old man who lives in Halifax with his wife. He currently works at a wholesaler as inventory specialist. He started that job 3 years ago. Lately he received a letter of warning because of poor work performance.

Chief Complaint Patient came to the office complaining of the following symptoms: poor attention, anxiety attacks, low energy, low libido, excessive worry, and irritability.

History of Present Illness Patient reported good mood and good appetite. He enjoys watching soccer and follows Manchester United Football team on TV. He also enjoys outdoor activities and goes fishing with his wife. His sleep has always been poor. He has difficulty initiating sleep. He never had suicidal thoughts.

Recently he started having two panic episodes every week. He used to have panic episodes once a month but lately the frequency increased. He has fear of being

© Springer International Publishing Switzerland 2017
J. Sadek, *Clinician's Guide to Adult ADHD Comorbidities*,
DOI 10.1007/978-3-319-39794-8_7

inside elevators since he had a traumatic experience inside an elevator when he was a child. Now he would only use the stairs and avoid elevators.

He worries a lot about everything. He cannot control his anxiety. His worries prevent him from sleeping. He becomes irritable and stressed with any small incident. His neck is always tense and he was told by his wife to go for massage therapy because his muscles are always tense particularly after his mother's diagnosis with cancer.

Andrew drinks socially a glass of wine once a week. He never used street drugs. Screening for other symptoms of mental illness was unrevealing.

Medications   Currently takes rosuvastatine (Crestor) 40 mg daily for dyslipidemia and melatonin 5 mg at bedtime for sleep.

Medical History   Allergy to penicillin. He has been diagnosed with high cholesterol and had vasectomy 3 years ago.

Family History   Patient had two sisters. Older sister passed away with breast cancer complications. Parents are alive and live together. Father has early dementia.

Mother has been diagnosed with generalized anxiety disorder and has been recently diagnosed with breast cancer.

7.2   Personal History

Patient was born in Toronto, Canada. Family moved to Halifax when he was 8 years old. His mother was healthy and never used street drugs and did not smoke or drink alcohol while pregnant with him. He was delivered by cesarean section.

He had some speech delay until he was 3 years old. He did not do well in school. Teachers told his mother to have him checked for ADHD because he was talking excessively, was loud, and could not sit in his seat most of the classes. He failed grade 10 and went to summer school. He also failed math in grade 11 and 12 then went to community college and finished 1 year only.

Andrew had significant anxiety as a child. His parents separated for 1 year when he was 9 years old, and his anxiety significantly increased after that. He could not be away from his mother for any extended period. He had to call her many times during the day and when she was late, he would have a panic attack. He had a great need to be closer to his mother and she was very concerned about that so she arranged for him to see a child psychiatrist who diagnosed him with ADHD and anxiety. She refused to give him medication then but he had psychotherapy for anxiety and it helped him.

Anthony has many friends. He has been with his partner since he was 20 years old. He cheated on her twice but he never told her. They never had any children together.

Patient currently endorses the following ADHD symptoms: often does not seem to listen when spoken to directly, often looses things (ten bank cards in the past

2 years), often has difficulty sustaining attention in tasks. He cannot finish few pages of any book. He is often disorganized and his car and work space are extremely messy. He starts many projects but fails to finish them. He started painting his base-ment a year ago and never finished it. He is often forgetful in daily activities and requires reminders from his wife every day.

He often avoids tasks that require sustained attention such as doing his sales reports. His wife purchased melatonin for him from the drugstore to help him sleep. He feels that melatonin helped his sleep. Currently he does not endorse hyperactiv-ity impulsivity symptoms except for feeling restless all the time.

Impression and Plan   Generalized anxiety disorder, panic disorder, agoraphobia, and ADHD inattentive type.

Patient was started on atomoxetine (Strattera) 20 mg AM for 2 weeks then the dosage increased to 40 mg AM for 2 weeks. He was also given a prescription for ten tablets of lorazepam 0.5 mg to take in cases of panic attacks only. He returned for a follow up visit after 2 weeks and reported that he used only one of the lorazepam tablets and he tolerated atomoxetine very well.

He was also referred to a psychologist. In the second follow up visit, his anxiety symptoms and ADD symptoms were much improved. He found the medications very helpful.

He was able to have five psychotherapy sessions because this was the maximum number of sessions allowed by his insurance plan. Medication dose was titrated gradually up to 80 mg daily and he showed continued improvement in his symp-toms. Lorazepam was discontinued.

Literature Review Questions on ADHD and Anxiety
Describe the prevalence rates and epidemiological data of ADHD and anxiety?
The comorbidity rates of ADHD and anxiety have been estimated to be up to 50 % [1].

The following tables compare the rates of different anxiety disorders in patients with or without ADHD.

Canadian study [2]	Comorbidity rates in patients with ADHD	Comorbidity rates in patients without ADHD
Specific phobia	6 %	0.9 %
Social anxiety	11 %	4.5 %
Panic disorder	6.6 %	2.7 %
American study [1]	Comorbidity rates in patients with ADHD	Comorbidity rates in patients without ADHD
Specific phobia	22.7 %	7.8 %
Social anxiety	9.5	8.9 %
Panic disorder	29.3 %	3.1 %
Any comorbid anxiety disorder	47.1 %	19.5 %

What are the overlapping and differentiating symptoms between ADHD and anxiety?

	Overlapping symptoms	Differentiating symptoms
GAD	Difficulty concentrating and distractibility Restlessness Onset of symptoms are common in childhood	Excessive anxiety and worries that the patient finds difficult to control and is associated with symptoms such as easily fatigued, muscle tension, irritability, and sleep disturbance
PTSD	Problems with concentration and attention, reckless behavior, memory complaint Cause significant distress or impairment in social, academic, occupational, or any important area of functioning	The intrusive re-experiencing of the traumatic events Avoidance of reminders of traumatic events and negative cognition and mood that characterize PTSD. The memory problems are specific to inability to remember important aspects of traumatic events
Panic	Decrease concentration and attention Cause significant distress or impairment in social, academic, occupational, or any important area of functioning	Presence of recurrent panic attacks with physical symptoms such as palpitations, sweating, trembling, chills, or cognitive symptoms Worry about having additional panic attacks
Agoraphobia	Decrease concentration and cause significant distress or impairment in social, academic, occupational, or any important area of functioning	Fear or anxiety of being in public places, enclosed places, using public transportation, standing in line or with a crowed, or being home alone
Social anxiety	Decrease concentration and attention Cause significant distress or impairment in social, academic, occupational, or any important area of functioning	The anxiety is about social situations and the focus is on fear of being negatively evaluated by others
OCD (separate category)	Decrease concentration and attention Cause significant distress or impairment in social, academic, occupational, or any important area of functioning	Presence of obsessions, compulsions, or both

(Kooij et al. [3]; APA [4])

Describe some of the difficulties in conducting meta-analysis on the effect of stimulant medications on comorbid anxiety in ADHD patients in the current literature?

Meta-analysis for the effect of stimulant medication on anxiety has been difficult to conduct for several reasons such as the use of different rating scales, different reporting methods, having no numerical results obtained or reported on rating scales, and reporting on partial findings only.

List some of the instruments that would assist clinicians in identifying different anxiety disorders?

Disorder	Scale	References
Generalized anxiety disorder	7-item Hamilton Rating Scale	[5]
OCD	Yale-Brown Obsessive Compulsive Scale	[6]
PTSD	PTSD Checklist	[7]
Social anxiety	Liebowitz Social Anxiety Scale	[8]
Panic disorder	Panic Appraisal Inventory	[9]
Phobia	Fear Questionnaire	[10]

What are the treatment considerations in comorbid ADHD and anxiety disorders?

Some authors raised concerns that stimulant medications may lead to exacerbation of anxiety disorders and sleep problems in patients with comorbid ADHD and anxiety disorders [11–13].

Some reports suggest that anxiety does not lessen response to ADHD stimulant treatment [14].

Combinations of SSRI and stimulant medications have been combined successfully in the management of both conditions [15, 16].

Atomoxetine was found to be efficacious in reducing ADHD and anxiety symptoms in patients who had both conditions [17].

Multiple studies demonstrate the efficacy of a cognitive-behavioral therapy intervention (CBT) in the treatment of OCD, ADHD, or comorbid anxiety disorders in both adults and adolescents. Nonpharmacological, psychosocial intervention may be a useful adjunct to pharmacotherapy in patients with ADHD and anxiety [18, 19].

Some guidelines recommend treating the most disabling disorder first. If clinicians start with ADHD treatment with a stimulant medication and the anxiety symptoms increase, then stimulant medication should be decreased or discontinued. Combination of SSRIs and stimulant medications are possible but frequent monitoring is required [20].

References

1. Kessler RC, Adler L, Barkley R et al (2006) The prevalence and correlates of adult ADHD in the United States: results from the National Comorbidity Survey Replication. Am J Psychiatry 163(4):716–723
2. Cumyn L, French L, Hechtman L (2009) Comorbidity in adults with attention deficit hyperactivity disorder. Can J Psychiatry 54(10):673–683
3. Kooij JJ, Huss M, Asherson P et al (2012) Distinguishing comorbidity and successful management of adult ADHD. J Atten Disord 16(5 suppl):3S–19S
4. American Psychiatric Association (2013) Diagnostic and statistical manual of mental disorders, 5th edn. American Psychiatric Association, Washington, DC

5. Spitzer RL, Kroenke K et al (2006) A brief measure for assessing generalized anxiety disorder: the GAD–7. Arch Intern Med 166(10):1092–1097
6. Tan O, Metin B, Metin S (2016) Obsessive-compulsive adults with and without childhood ADHD symptoms. Atten Defic Hyperact Disord. [Epub ahead of print] PubMed PMID: 27056070
7. Ford JD, Connor DF (2009) ADHD and posttraumatic stress disorder. Current Atten Disord Rep 1(2):60–66
8. Tyrala K, Seweryn M, Bonk M, Bulska W, Orszulak K, Bratek A, Krysta K (2015) Evaluation of the utility of Liebowitz Social Anxiety Scale and Barratt Impulsiveness Scale in the diagnosis of social anxiety, impulsivity and depression. Psychiatr Danub 27(Suppl 1):S223–S226
9. Schulte-van Maaren YW, Giltay EJ, van Hemert AM, Zitman FG, de Waal MW, Carlier IV (2013) Reference values for anxiety questionnaires: the Leiden Routine Outcome Monitoring Study. J Affect Disord 150(3):1008–1018
10. Marks IM (1979) Mathews: brief standard self-rating for phobic patients. Behav Res Ther 17:263–267
11. Duong S, Chung K, Wigal SB (2012) Metabolic, toxicological, and safety considerations for drugs used to treat ADHD. Expert Opin Drug Metab Toxicol 8(5):543–552
12. Pliszka SR (1989) Effect of anxiety on cognition, behavior, and stimulant response in ADHD. J Am Acad Child Adolesc Psychiatry 28:882–887
13. van der Oord S, Prins PJ, Oosterlaan J et al (2008) Treatment of attention deficit hyperactivity disorder in children: predictors of treatment outcome. Eur Child Adolesc Psychiatry 17:73–81
14. Abikoff H, McGough J, Vitiello B, McCracken J, Davies M, Walkup J, Riddle M, Oatis M, Greenhill L, Skrobala A, March J, Gammon P, Robinson J, Lazell R, McMahon DJ, Ritz L (2005) RUPP ADHD/Anxiety Study Group. Sequential pharmacotherapy for children with comorbid attention-deficit/hyperactivity and anxiety disorders. J Am Acad Child Adolesc Psychiatry. 44(5):418–427.
15. Lavretsky H, Reinlieb M, St Cyr N, Siddarth P, Ercoli LM, Senturk D (2015) Citalopram, methylphenidate, or their combination in geriatric depression: a randomized, double-blind, placebo-controlled trial. Am J Psychiatry 172(6):561–569
16. Koran LM, Aboujaoude E, Gamel NN (2009) Double-blind study of dextroamphetamine versus caffeine augmentation for treatment-resistant obsessive-compulsive disorder. J Clin Psychiatry 70(11):1530–1535
17. Adler LA, Liebowitz M, Kronenberger W et al (2009) Atomoxetine treatment in adults with attention-deficit/hyperactivity disorder and comorbid social anxiety disorder. Depress Anxiety 26(3):212–221
18. Antshel KM, Faraone SV, Gordon M (2014) Cognitive behavioral treatment outcomes in adolescent ADHD. J Atten Disord 18(6):483–495
19. Houghton S, Alsalmi N, Tan C, Taylor M, Durkin K (2013) Treating Comorbid Anxiety in Adolescents With ADHD Using a Cognitive Behavior Therapy Program Approach. J Atten Disord. [Epub ahead of print] PubMed PMID: 23382576.
20. www.CADDRA.ca

Bibliography

Childress AC (2015) A critical appraisal of atomoxetine in the management of ADHD. Ther Clin Risk Manag 12:27–39

Appendix A: Sadek ADHD Checklist (SAC)©

	Symptom of Inattention: Mnemonic: Details Off	Never	Rarely	Sometimes	Often	Very often
D	**DETAILS** often missed or makes careless mistakes *in schoolwork, work, other activities*					
E	**EASILY distracted** by stimuli *(e.g. noise, movement, day dream a lot)*					
TA	**TASK AVOIDANCE** *(that requires attention such as homework, completing reports, forms)*					
I	**INSTRUCTIONS** missed because mind elsewhere Or not listening when spoken to directly					
L	**LOSE** things (e.g. wallet, keys, books, toy, homework)					
S	**SUSTAINING attention** is problematic *(during reading, lectures or other activities)*					
O	**ORGANIZATIONAL problems** *(messy, disorganized work, difficulty organizing time)*					
F	**Fails to FINISH** activities, schoolwork, chores or duties in the workplace or not following through on instructions.					
F	**FORGETFUL** in daily activities *(e.g. doing homework, remembering appointments, paying bills)*					
	(Often or very often) Total Adults 5/9					

© Springer International Publishing Switzerland 2017
J. Sadek, *Clinician's Guide to Adult ADHD Comorbidities*,
DOI 10.1007/978-3-319-39794-8

		Total Children 6/9					
		Symptoms of Hyperactivity Impulsivity **Mnemonic: RAPID GIRL**					
R	**RUNS** about or climbs excessively in inappropriate situation/or **Restlessness** feeling a lot of the time						
A	**ANSWERS blurted** before question is complete or blurt out rude comments						
P	**PLENTY of talk** in social situation or play						
I	**INTERRUPTS OR INTRUDES on others** (e.g. butts in conversations or games,)						
D	**DIFFICULTY awaiting turn** (e.g. waiting to speak in turn, waiting on line, cut through traffic)						
G	**GOING non stop** or cannot unwind and relax						
I	**IMPATIENCE** with prolonged seating (leaves seat in classroom or long meeting)						
R	**RESTLESS**; always fidgets or squirms (e.g. taps legs or fingers)						
L	**LOUD** or noisy						
		Total adults 5/9					
		Total children 6/9					

List of Scales: Adults

- *Adult Self Report Scale (ASRS)*: This is based on self-report of current symptoms and has a long version with 18 items and short version with 6 items. Symptom frequency is based on a five-point Likert scale (0–4). The six items with the most stable psychometric properties were chosen for the short ASRS.
- *Adult Rating Scale (ARS)*: This is based on self and informant report of childhood and current symptoms with 25 items using Likert scale (0–3). The items are derived from the DSM-III-R criteria, and is of similar format to the children's version of this scale.

- *ADHD Rating Scale (ADHD-RS)*: This is based on self and informant report of childhood and current symptoms. This is a self-reporting scale with a long (18 items – 9 inattention, 9 hyperactivity) and short version (6 items) of current symptoms using a Likert scale (0–3). Criteria used: DSM-IV.
- *Attention Deficit Scales for Adults (ADSA)*: This is a self-reporting scale of current symptoms with 54 items using a five-point rating (1–5). Answers are recorded on an answer sheet. This scale was developed based on clinical experience and is divided into nine subscales: attention, interpersonal, disorganization, coordination, academic theme, emotive, long term, childhood, and negative social elements. Additionally an inconsistency index is included.
- *Adult Problems Questionnaire (APQ)*: This is a self-reporting scale of current symptoms with 43 items (score range 0–3) that includes the common symptoms of ADHD adults. The questions are based on the DSM-IV and the Utah criteria.
- *Assessment of Hyperactivity and Attention (AHA)*: This is both a self-reporting and informant rating scale of current and childhood symptoms. Eighteen items rate based on DSM-IV criteria. Here answers are given with a "yes" or "no" reply, and two subscales are covered including inattention and hyperactivity.
- *Brown Attention Deficit Disorder Scales (BADDS)*: This 40-item self-reporting scale of current symptoms is divided into five subscales, those being organization/work, attention, energy/effort, mood, and memory. A scoring sheet is used for answering. Items are based on DSM-IV criteria, as well as based on the author's clinical observations and several studies.
- *Current Symptoms Scale (CSS)*: Another self-reporting scale with two subscales of nine items each on inattention and hyperactivity/impulsivity. Rating on a 0–3 Likert scale, the items are specifically from the DSM-IV "A" criteria. It has been used for retrospective childhood symptom report.
- *Conners Adult ADHD Rating Scale (CAARS)*: There is both a long and short version of this rating scale (66 long, 26 short) and can be completed by the patient or someone else reporting current symptoms. This scale was developed from the children's version and the Utah criteria of nine domains. T scores between 50 and 65 are considered borderline and require interpretation by a trained clinician.
- *Symptom Inventory (SI)*: An 18-scale self-report of current symptoms broken down into two subscales: inattention and hyperactivity/impulsivity. This was developed for use in the developers' clinic based on the DSM-IV criteria.
- *Wender Utah ADHD Rating Scale (WURS)*: The WURS includes a long (61 item) and short (25 item) self-reporting scale that includes current and childhood symptoms. Items were taken from Wender's *Minimal Brain Dysfunction in Children*. The short version can also be reported by other than patient informant. It has robust psychometric properties. Symptom frequency is based on a five-point Likert scale (0–4).
- *Young Adults Questionnaire (YAQ)*: This is a 112-item scale for self-reporting of childhood symptoms. There are four subscales (ADHD symptoms, emotional delinquency, and social environments). This scale was developed based on a literature review of ADHD symptoms and comorbid factors.
- *Young Adult Rating Scale (YARS)*: Here 24 items mostly all based on DSM-IV criteria report an individual's current symptoms, including those experienced during college.

Appendix B: Adult ADHD Self-Report Scale (ASRS-v.1.1)

For an up-to-date copy of this scale please refer to: http://www.hcp.med.harvard.edu/ncs/asrs.php

Adult ADHD Self-Report Scale (ASRS-v1.1) Symptom Checklist

Patient Name		Today's Date					
Please answer the questions below, rating yourself on each of the criteria shown using the scale on the right side of the page. As you answer each question, place an X in the box that best describes how you have felt and conducted yourself over the past 6 months. Please give this completed checklist to your healthcare professional to discuss during today's appointment.			Never	Rarely	Sometimes	Often	Very Often
1. How often do you have trouble wrapping up the final details of a project, once the challenging parts have been done?							
2. How often do you have difficulty getting things in order when you have to do a task that requires organization?							
3. How often do you have problems remembering appointments or obligations?							
4. When you have a task that requires a lot of thought, how often do you avoid or delay getting started?							
5. How often do you fidget or squirm with your hands or feet when you have to sit down for a long time?							
6. How often do you feel overly active and compelled to do things, like you were driven by a motor?							
							Part A
7. How often do you make careless mistakes when you have to work on a boring or difficult project?							
8. How often do you have difficulty keeping your attention when you are doing boring or repetitive work?							
9. How often do you have difficulty concentrating on what people say to you, even when they are speaking to you directly?							
10. How often do you misplace or have difficulty finding things at home or at work?							
11. How often are you distracted by activity or noise around you?							
12. How often do you leave your seat in meetings or other situations in which you are expected to remain seated?							
13. How often do you feel restless or fidgety?							
14. How often do you have difficulty unwinding and relaxing when you have time to yourself?							
15. How often do you find yourself talking too much when you are in social situations?							
16. When you're in a conversation, how often do you find yourself finishing the sentences of the people you are talking to, before they can finish them themselves?							
17. How often do you have difficulty waiting your turn in situations when turn taking is required?							
18. How often do you interrupt others when they are busy?							
							Part B

Adult ADHD Self-Report Scale (ASRS v1.1)

Symptoms Checklist Instructions

The questions for the ASRS are designed to stimulate dialogue between you and your patients and to help confirm if they may be suffering from the symptoms of attention-deficit hyperactivity disorder (ADHD).

Description
The Symptom Checklist is an instrument consisting of the 18 DSM-IV-TR criteria. Six of the 18 questions were found to be the most predictive of symptoms consistent with ADHD. These six questions are the basis for the ASRS v1.1 Screener and are also Part A of the Symptom Checklist. Part B of the Symptom Checklist contains the remaining 12 questions.

Instructions
Symptoms
1. Ask the patient to complete both Part A and Part B of the Symptom Checklist by marking an x in the box that most closely represents the frequency of occurrence of each of the symptoms.
2. Score Part A. If four or more marks appear in the darkly shaded boxes within Part A then the patient has symptoms highly consistent with ADHD in adults and further investigation is warranted.
3. The frequency scores on Part B provide additional cues and can serve as further probes into the patient's symptoms. Pay particular attention to marks appearing in the dark shaded boxes. The frequency-based response is more sensitive with certain questions. No total score or diagnostic likelihood is utilized for the 12 questions. It has been found that the six questions in Part A are the most predictive of the disorder and are best for use as a screening instrument.

Impairments
1. Review the entire Symptom Checklist with your patients and evaluate the level of impairment associated with the symptom.
2. Consider work/school, social and family settings.
3. Symptom frequency is often associated with symptom severity, therefore the Symptom Checklist may also aid in the assessment of impairments. If your patients have frequent symptoms, you may want to ask them to describe how these problems have affected the ability to work, take care of things at home, or get along with other people such as their spouse/significant other.

History
1. Assess the presence of these symptoms or similar symptoms in childhood. Adults who have ADHD need not have been formally diagnosed on childhood. In evaluating a patient's history, look for evidence of early-appearing and long-standing problems with attention or self-control. Some significant symptoms should have been present in childhood, but full symptomology is not necessary.

The Value of Screening for Adults with ADHD

Research suggests that the symptoms of ADHD can persist into adulthood, having a significant impact on relationships, careers, and even the personal safety of your patients who may suffer from it [1–4]. Because this disorder is often misunderstood, many people who have it do not receive appropriate treatment and, as a result, may never reach their full potential. Part of the problem is that it can be difficult to diagnose, particularly in adults.

The Adult ADHD Self-Report Scale (ASRS-v1.1) Symptom Checklist was developed in conjunction with the World Health Organization (WHO), and the Workgroup on Adult ADHD that included the following team of psychiatrists and researchers:

- Lenard Adler, MD, Associate Professor of Psychiatry and Neurology
- Ronald C. Kessler, PhD, Professor, Department of Health Care Policy, Harvard Medical School
- Thomas Spencer, MD, Associate Professor of Psychiatry, Harvard Medical School

As the healthcare professional, you can use the ASRS v1.1 as a tool to help screen for ADHD in adult patients. Insights gained through this screening may suggest the need for a more in-depth clinician review. The questions in the ASRS v1.1 are consistent with DSM-IV criteria and address the manifestations of ADHD symptoms in adults. Content of the questionnaire also reflects the importance that DSM-IV places on symptoms, impairments, and history for a correct diagnosis (American Psychiatric Association 2000).

The checklist takes about minutes to complete and can provide information that is critical to supplement the diagnostic process.

References

American Psychiatric Association (2000) Diagnostic manual of mental disorders, 4th edn. American Psychiatric Association, Washington DC, pp 85–93

Barkley RA (1998) Attention deficit hyperactivity disorder: a handbook for diagnostic and treatment, 2nd edn. Guilford Press, New York

Biederman J et al (1993) Patterns of psychiatric comorbidity, cognition, and psychosocial functioning in adults with attention deficit hyperactivity disorder. Am J Psychiatry 150: 1792–1798

Schweitzer JB et al (2001) Attention-deficit/hyperactivity disorder. Med Clin North Am 85(3): 10–11, 757–777

For up-to-date copy of this scale please refer to: http://www.hcp.med.harvard.edu/ncs/asrs.php

Appendix C: Sadek ADHD Differential Diagnosis©

Conditions that can mimic ADHD	Symptoms or signs not characteristic of ADHD
Psychiatric disorders	
Generalized anxiety disorder	Worry for 6 months or more that the person cannot control, lack of energy, anxious mood and somatic anxiety symptoms
Obsessive compulsive disorder	Presence of obsessions or compulsions that interfere with level of function
Major depression	Episodic change from baseline, depressed, or irritable mood during an episode; suicide-related issues; low energy; psychomotor retardation
Bipolar disorder I or II (manic or hypomanic episode)	Episodic change from baseline, psychotic symptoms, grandiosity, pressured speech, recent decreased need for sleep
Psychotic disorder (schizophrenia or schizoaffective disorder)	Psychotic symptoms
Pervasive developmental disorder	Qualitative impairment in social interactions, communication, or odd eccentric behaviors
Oppositional defiant disorder	Defiant, loses temper, annoys others, and is easily annoyed; spiteful or vindictive
Conduct disorder	Presence of conduct disorder criteria, e.g., aggression to people and animals, destruction of property, deceitfulness or theft, serious violations of rules
Substance abuse	Urine toxicology screen confirms presence of substance Signs and symptoms of intoxication or withdrawal
Learning disorder	Testing and consultation with learning disorder specialist confirms presence of the disorder
Language disorder	Testing and consultation with speech-language specialist confirms presence of the disorder
Tic disorder/Tourette syndrome	Presence of vocal or motor tics or both
Personality disorders	
Borderline personality disorder	Abandonment anxiety, hourly mood fluctuations, suicidal threats or behavior, identity disturbance, dissociative symptoms, or micro psychotic episodes; chronic feelings of emptiness

Conditions that can mimic ADHD	Symptoms or signs not characteristic of ADHD
Antisocial personality disorder	Lack of remorse, lack of responsibility, lack of empathy, deceitfulness, and aggression
IQ-related problems: Intellectual disability Gifted child	Cognitive assessment confirms diagnosis Note: IQ within the normal range: explore if curriculum is not well matched to child's ability
Medication-related	
Mood stabilizers with cognitive dulling side effect	
Decongestants or beta agonist with psychomotor activation	
General medical condition	Investigations confirm the diagnosis of the medical condition
Head trauma/concussion	Since underlying ADHD can increase risk for head trauma, it is important to look for timing of cognitive symptoms apparition (present before, or appeared or worsened after head trauma)
Seizure disorders	Neurology assessment confirms diagnosis
Tic disorder/Tourette syndrome	Presence of vocal or motor tics
Hearing impairment or vision impairment	Audition and vision evaluation confirms diagnosis
Thyroid dysfunction	TSH levels indicate hypothyroidism or hyperthyroidism
Hypoglycemia	Abnormally low glucose blood levels confirm diagnosis
Severe anemia	CBC and anemia investigations confirm diagnosis
Lead poisoning	Lead blood level measurement confirms diagnosis
Sleep disorders	Sleep lab assessment confirms diagnosis
Fragile X syndrome	Genotype confirms diagnosis
Fetal alcohol syndrome	Molecular genetic testing for FMRI gene confirms diagnosis. Possible presence of mental retardation
Phenylketonuria	Blood test confirms diagnosis
Neurofibromatosis	Café au lait spots
Other factors	
Unsafe or disruptive learning environment	
Family dysfunction or poor parenting	
Child abuse or neglect	
Attachment disorder	

Appendix D: Comorbid Problems That Can Complicate ADHD Evaluation and Management©

Psychiatric problems	Evaluation considerations	Pharmacological management consideration	Psychosocial management consideration problems
Depression	Questions about suicide must be a priority and should not be ignored	ADHD medications might be less effective in depressed patients	Psychological treatment for depression is not part of ADHD management. Do both
Bipolar mania	Diagnosis of ADHD should not be made while patient is manic	Treatment of ADHD can be offered when bipolar disorder is stabilized. Consider drug-drug interactions	Psychosocial treatment for ADHD is very important because some patients cannot tolerate ADHD medications
Schizophrenia or schizoaffective disorder	Diagnosis of ADHD should not be made while patient is psychotic	Avoid stimulant medication	Psychosocial treatment for ADHD is very important because some patients cannot tolerate ADHD medications
Substance use disorder (SUD)	Diagnosis of ADHD should not be made while patient is in state of intoxication or withdrawal	ADHD medications should be avoided if patient insists on the same level of substance or alcohol use	Motivational interview and psychosocial treatment for ADHD can be initiated early
Anxiety disorders	Careful clarifications of anxiety-related symptoms versus ADHD symptoms should be made	Combinations of stimulant medications and SNRI should be monitored carefully because of increased blood pressure	CBT for any of the anxiety disorders can be very helpful
Borderline personality disorder	List of BPD symptoms should be separated from ADHD symptoms	Be careful with the amount of prescription medications given since some patients may overdose on medications	Dialectical behavioral therapy for BPD can be helpful but do not ignore ADHD psychosocial issues

Psychiatric problems	Evaluation considerations	Pharmacological management consideration	Psychosocial management consideration problems
Antisocial personality disorder	Clarify the duration of ADHD symptoms versus the ASPD symptoms	Ensure that patients do not sell their medications	ADHD does not justify antisocial behaviors and patients should not expect that ADHD medication will cure the antisocial behavior

Appendix E: Stimulant Medications

Methylphenidate-based products		Amphetamine-based products	
MPH IR (Ritalin®) 10 and 20 mg tablets	• Start with 5 to 10 mg b.i.d. to t.i.d. • Increase by 5 to 10 mg weekly • Maximum dose 60 mg for children and adolescents and 60 mg for adults (some experts recommend higher doses).	**Dexedrine®** (Dextroamphetamine) 5 mg tablet	• Start with 2.5 to 5 mg b.i.d. • Increase by 5 mg weekly • Maximum dose 40 mg for children, adolescents and adults.
Ritalin® SR (MPH) 20 mg tablet	• Start with 20 mg in the morning • Increase by 20 mg weekly • **Maximum dose 60 mg for children and for adolescents and adults 60 mg (some experts recommend higher doses).	**Dexedrin® Spansule®** 10 and 15 mg spansule	• Start with 10 mg in the morning • Increase by 5 to 10 mg weekly • Maximum dose 40 mg for all ages.
Biphentin® 10, 15, 20, 30, 40, 50, 60, 70, 80 mg capsule (1ˢᵗ line)	• Start with 10 to 20 mg in the morning • Increase by 10 mg weekly • Maximum dose 60 mg for children and 80 mg for adolescents and adults. *40% immediate and 60% delayed release*	**Adderall XR®** (Amphetamine mixed salt) 5, 10, 15, 20, 25, 30 mg capsules (1ˢᵗ line) *Delivers 50% immediate and 50% delayed release*	• Start with 5 to 10 mg in the morning for children, 10 mg for adolescents and adults • Increase by 5 to 10 mg weekly • Maximum dose 30 mg for children and 30 mg for adolescents and adults.
Concerta® 18, 27, 36, 54 mg tablets (1ˢᵗ line)	• Start with 18 mg in the morning • Increase by 18 mg weekly • Maximum dose 54 mg for children, 54 mg for adolescents, and 72 mg for adults.	**Vyvanse®** (Lisdexamfetamine dimesylate) 20, 30, 40, 50, 60 mg capsules (1st line)	• Start with 20 to 30 mg in the morning • Increase by 10 mg weekly • Maximum dose 60 mg for children and 70 mg for adolescents and adults.
MPH ER-C 18, 27, 36, 54 mg tablet	• Start with 18 mg in the morning • Increase by 18 mg weekly • Maximum dose 54 mg for all ages according to product monograph		

Websites

ADHD Guidelines Available on the Internet:

Canadian ADHD Guidelines: http://www.caddra.ca/cms4/
American Psychological Association: http://www.apa.org/topics/adhd/index.aspx
Scottish ADHD Guidelines: http://www.sign.ac.uk/guidelines/fulltext/112/index.
html
National Institute for Health and Clinical Excellence NICE: http://publications.
nice.org.uk/attention-deficit-hyperactivity-disorder-cg72
Australian ADHD Draft Guidelines: http://www.nhmrc.gov.au/guidelines/publica-
tions/ch54

Other Websites of Interest:

A ADDitude: Living well with Attention Deficit Magazine http://www.addi-
tudemag.com
B ADDvance: Answers to Your Questions about ADD (ADHD) http://www.
addvance.com
C American Academy of Child and Adolescent Psychiatry (AACAP) http://www.
aacap.org
D American Academy of Family Physicians (AAFP) http://www.aafp.org/online/
en/home.html
E American Academy of Pediatrics (AAP) http://www.aap.org and http://www.
healthychildren.org
F American Association of People with Disabilities (AAPD) http://www.aapd.
com
G American Medical Association (AMA) http://www.ama-assn.org
H Attention Deficit Disorder Association (ADDA) http://www.add.org
I CADDRA http://www.caddra.ca
J Centre for Disease Control http://www.cdc.gov/ncbddd/actearly/pdf/parents_
pdfs/adhdfactsheet.pdf
K Children and Adults with Attention Deficit/Hyperactivity Disorder (HADD)
http://www.chadd.org
L Consortium for Citizens with Disabilities (CCD) http://www.c-c-d.org/
M Council for Learning Disabilities (CLD) http://www.cldinternational.org/
N Internet Mental Health http://www.mentalhealth.com/
O Learning Disabilities Association of America (LDA) http://www.ldanatl.org/
P Lives in the Balance http://www.livesinthebalance.org/
Q National Dissemination Center for Children with Disabilities (NICHCY) http://
nichcy.org/
R National Alliance on Mental Illness http://www.nami.org/
S National Clearing House http://www.help4adhd.org/

T National Institute of Mental Health (NIMH) http://www.nimh.nih.gov/health/topics/attention-deficit-hyperactivity-disorder-adhd/index.shtml

U Northern County Psychiatric Association http://www.ncpamd.com/

V Parent Advocacy Coalition for Educational Rights (PACER) Center http://www.pacer.org/

W Substance Abuse & Mental Health Services Administration (SAMHSA) http://www.samhsa.gov/

Appendix F: ADHD Medication Adverse Effects and How to Manage Them

Tics	Growth and appetite suppression
◉ Tic Disorder is not a contraindication for psychostimulant use; however, several patients may suffer from worsening of tics. ◉ Taking a history, and closely monitoring comorbid tics is needed. ◉ *Tics are naturally waxing and waning. It is often difficult to decide if worsening of tics is provoked by the ADHD medication.* ◉ *May add antipsychotic to the stimulant or Atomoxetine.* ◉ *The alpha-2 adrenergic agonist Clonidine and Guanfacine have been showing promise in the treatment of tics, particularly in combination with stimulant medications.*	• Monitor growth (weight and height) closely and use the growth charts in children ◉ Consuming additional meals, or snacks, early in the morning or late in the evening when the stimulant effects of the drug have worn off; ◉ Obtaining dietary advice ◉ Consuming high calorie foods; ◉ Changing the timing of the dose and/or meals ; ◉ Consuming high energy snacks ◉ The option of a planned break in treatment over school holidays may be considered to allow "catch-up" growth to occur. Drug holidays can be planned. ◉ If there is evidence of weight loss associated with drug treatment in adults with ADHD, clinicians should consider monitoring body mass index and changing the drug if weight loss persists. ◉ In children, follow the medical criteria for referral to pediatric endocrinologist to consider growth hormone therapy in treatment of short stature, particularly if the height is more than 2 standard deviations below the population mean for the age, and a one year decrease of more than .5 standard deviation in height. ◉ Consideration should also be given to the mother and father's height.
	Jaundice, signs of liver disease
	◉ Stop medication immediately ◉ Consult a specialist
	Psychotic Symptoms
	◉ A full psychiatric assessment should be conducted to determine if the psychotic symptoms are primary or secondary. ◉ A determination of starting AP should be made at that point.

Sleep Disturbance	Suicide
◉ Some clinicians concluded from several studies that the effect of ADHD medication on sleep may be beneficial, at least in some patients, but further research with more subjects, and with a variety of medication, is needed. ◉ Many patients treated with psychostimulants complain of insomnia, so an approach to manage this problem is necessary. ◉ Document sleep patterns and complaints before treatment ◉ Sleep hygiene, consisting of simple behavioral approaches that promote sound sleep (e.g., creating a restful environment and avoiding caffeine), is a primary approach for most patients with insomnia. ◉ Look into shifting the dose to an earlier time or reducing an existing evening dose. ◉ Mirtazapine 15 mg HS has been reported as safe and effective for adults taking psychostimulants. ◉ Atomoxetine may have an effect on sleep that is different from that of psychostimulants, including reduced sleep latency, but less efficiency ◉ Melatonin 3 to 6 mg at least half hour before sleep can be used. ◉ Other options inclu de: ◉ Zopiclone 7.5 mg HS ◉ Trazodone 25 to 50 mg HS ◉ Benzodiazepines, such as Lorazepam, (consider the high addiction potential), ◉ Methotrimeprazine 10 to 15 mg HS, or Quetiapine 25 mg HS for some resistant cases.	◉ First, assess the suicide as a separate issue. Determine whether the patient is expressing suicidal ideation, intent, plan or is there a history of chronic self-harm behavior as in a personality disorder. ◉ Evaluate if suicide developed after starting ADHD medications or part of a mood disorder or personality disorder. ◉ Suicide prevention should be the first priority over any other consideration. Families and caregivers should be advised of the need to recognize any emergence of emotional change, or self-injurious thinking, and to communicate well with the prescriber. ◉ If SI do emerge in treatment, consideration should be given to dose reduction and/or other changes in therapeutic regimen, including the possibility of discontinuing medication, especially if symptoms are severe or abrupt in onset, or were not part of the patient's presenting symptoms. ◉ Treat co morbid disorders.
Cardiovascular adverse effects (monitor closely and consider consulting specialist)	Seizure (treat with anticonvulsant)

Appendix G: Sadek Assessment Tool of Suicidality (SATS)©

Sadek assessment Tool of suicidality (SATS) ©

Date _____ Time _____ Assessor _____ Diagnosis _____

Reason: ☐ MH Assessment ☐ Admission/Transfer/Discharge ☐ Acute deterioration_____

Interview Risk Profile	Individual Risk Profile	Risk Buffers – Not to be used to determine degree of risk.
☐ Suicidal thinking or Ideation	☐ Ethnic risk group or refugee	
☐ Access to lethal means	☐ Family history of suicide	☐ Has reason to live/hope
☐ Suicide intent or lethal plan or plan for after death (note)	☐ Trauma: as domestic violence / sexual abuse/neglect	☐ Social support
☐ Hopelessness	☐ Poor self-control: impulsive / violent/aggression	☐ Responsibility for family/kids/pets
☐ Intense Emotions: rage, anger, agitation, humiliation, revenge, panic, severe anxiety	☐ Recent suicide attempt	☐ Capacity to cope/resilience
		☐ Religion/ faith
	☐ Other past suicide attempts, esp. with low rescue potential	☐ Strength for managing risk
☐ Current Alcohol or Substance intoxication/problematic use	☐ Mental illness or addiction	**Communication Plan**
☐ Withdrawing from family, friends	☐ Depression/ anhedonia	Verbal (V) Written/fax (W)
	☐ Psychotic	☐ Nurse:
☐ Poor Reasoning/Judgment	☐ Command hallucinations	☐ Physician:
☐ Clinical Intuition: assessor concerned	☐ Recent admission / discharge / ED visits	☐ SDM/Family:
		☐ Mobile Crisis:
☐ Recent Dramatic Change in mood	☐ Chronic medical illness/ pain	☐ Others:
	☐ Disability or impairment	
☐ Recent Crisis/Conflict/ Loss	☐ Collateral information supports suicide intent	☐ Documentation in chart
		Management Plan
Illness Management	**Circle of support**	☐ Regular outpatient follow-up
☐ Lack of clinical support	☐ Lack of family/ friends support	☐ Removal of lethal means
☐ Non compliance or poor response to treatment	☐ Caregiver unavailable	☐ Urgent outpatient follow-up
	☐ Frequent change of home	☐ Admission to a psychiatric unit
		o Routine observation
		o Close observation q 15 m
		o Constant observation

Suicide Risk Level: Risk assessment is based on clinical judgment and not based on number of items checked. The checklist is intended to guide the clinical decision only.

RISK LEVEL: ☐ **High**   ☐ **Moderate**   ☐ **Low**   Signature:_____

Analysis of Risk, Commentsand Collateral Information: _____

_____

_____

_____

_____

_____

For information about this form contact Dr. Joseph Sadek at joseph.sadek@nshealth.ca

Disclaimer

The text in this book, and its references, are for education, guidance, and information purposes only. Responsibility remains in the hands of the clinician diagnosing and treating their own patient to determine the correct course for their patient. No one who took part in creating this text can be held legally responsible for any of the information contained in the text.

© Springer International Publishing Switzerland 2017
J. Sadek, *Clinician's Guide to Adult ADHD Comorbidities*,
DOI 10.1007/978-3-319-39794-8

Printed in the United States
By Bookmasters